the**facts**

Epilepsy

THIRD EDITION

RICHARD E. APPLETON

Consultant Paediatric Neurologist
The Roald Dahl EEG Department
Paediatric Neurosciences Foundation
Alder Hey Children's NHS Foundation Trust
Liverpool.

ANTHONY G. MARSON

Consultant Neurologist
The Walton Centre for Neurology and
Neurosurgery, Liverpool.
Reader in Neurology
The University of Liverpool.

OXFORD
UNIVERSITY PRESS

OXFORD

UNIVERSITY PRESS

Great Clarendon Street, Oxford OX2 6DP

Oxford University Press is a department of the University of Oxford.
It furthers the University's objective of excellence in research, scholarship,
and education by publishing worldwide in

Oxford New York

Auckland Cape Town Dar es Salaam Hong Kong Karachi
Kuala Lumpur Madrid Melbourne Mexico City Nairobi
New Delhi Shanghai Taipei Toronto

With offices in

Argentina Austria Brazil Chile Czech Republic France Greece
Guatemala Hungary Italy Japan Poland Portugal Singapore
South Korea Switzerland Thailand Turkey Ukraine Vietnam

Oxford is a registered trade mark of Oxford University Press
in the UK and in certain other countries

Published in the United States
by Oxford University Press Inc., New York

British Library Cataloguing in Publication Data

Data available

Library of Congress Cataloguing-in-Publication Data

Appleton, Richard, 1995-Epilepsy, the facts / Richard Appleton, Anthony G.
Marson.—3rd ed.
  p.cm.—(The facts)
Includes index.
ISBN 978-0-19-923368-7
  1. Epilepsy—Popular works. 2. Epilepsy in children—Popular works.
I. Marson, Anthony G. II. Title.
RC372.A74 2008
616.8'53—dc22

2008036484

Typeset by Cepha Imaging Pvt. Ltd.,
Bangalore, India
Printed in China through
Asia Pacific Offset

ISBN 978-0-19-923368-7

10 9 8 7 6 5 4 3 2 1

Whilst every effort has been made to ensure that the contents of this book are as complete, accurate
and up-to-date as possible at the date of writing, Oxford University Press is not able to give any
guarantee or assurance that such is the case. Readers are urged to take appropriately qualified
medical advice in all cases. The information in this book is intended to be useful to the general
reader, but should not be used as a means of self-diagnosis or for the prescription of medication.

Epilepsy

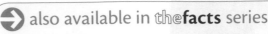
also available in the**facts** series

Foreword

Epilepsy is a condition that is still surrounded by mystery. Although attitudes towards the condition have improved over recent years, people with epilepsy still face prejudice and misunderstanding in many aspects of their daily lives. A book that increases people's knowledge of the condition is to be welcomed.

Epilepsy is a vast subject and a book of this size can't hope to cover every aspect. Despite its relatively modest size, *Epilepsy: The Facts* manages to pack in plenty of information. Not only are some of the more usual topics covered, but also less common ones, such as rare epilepsy syndromes. Although febrile seizures are not classified as epilepsy, it's good to find such comprehensive information here, as it is often difficult to find elsewhere.

People with epilepsy often tell us that they feel their own experiences of living with epilepsy are not listened to, so it is particularly good to see included a first-hand account of living with epilepsy from Sam, a teenager with epilepsy, and his parents.

Many books are available on epilepsy. Some only give the most basic information. Others are so technical that only an epilepsy specialist can understand them. *Epilepsy: The Facts* is different. Yes, there is a lot of medical information, as you would expect from two eminent epilepsy professionals, but the book is most definitely written for the non-specialist.

Epilepsy Action's vision is to live in a society where everyone understands epilepsy and where attitudes towards the condition are based on fact not fiction. This book is a very useful contribution towards the realization of this vision.

Shelley Wagstaff
Epilepsy Action

Oxford University Press wishes to thank Shelley Wagstaff and all at Epilepsy Action for the invaluable (and considerable) time and effort put into the production of this book. We are extremely grateful for their help and suggestions.

Preface

Epilepsy, or, more appropriately, the epilepsies, is one of the most common groups of neurological disorders that may occur at any age, but most commonly start in childhood and in the elderly. Epilepsy is the name given to recurrent and usually unprovoked seizures (also known as 'fits' or 'attacks' or 'events'), of which the tonic–clonic convulsion is only one type. Just as there are many types of seizure, so are there many types of epilepsy, called 'epilepsy syndromes'. The identification of the different epilepsy syndromes is important because they have different causes, treatments and outcomes. There are also many causes of epilepsy including abnormal patterns of brain development, problems at birth, following head injuries and meningitis, genetic causes and rarely, brain tumours. However, in spite of major advances in methods of investigation, including detailed and sophisticated brain scans and genetic tests, an underlying cause will be found in just over one third of people of all ages with epilepsy.

Fortunately, over the last fifteen years or so, there has been significant progress in the treatment of the epilepsies with the development of many new anti-epileptic drugs (also known as anticonvulsants) that appear to be not only more effective but also safer than the older drugs. There are still more anti-epileptic drugs that are in the process of being developed. In addition, alternative treatments, including surgery and some diets have also become far more available during this time.

Undoubtedly we now know far more about the epilepsies than was known twelve years ago when the second edition of this book was published. This new information is relevant for anyone who has epilepsy, whatever their age and their sex and whether in school, college, employment or unemployment. This information has already resulted in a greater understanding of the epilepsies which has improved teachers', employers' and the general public's awareness and acceptance of the condition. However, much still needs to be done.

As has already been stated, epilepsy commonly starts in childhood and many of the epilepsies may continue throughout life. One of us is a paediatric neurologist and the other an adult neurologist and between us we have over thirty-five years of experience in looking after people with epilepsy; we also have a passion for the epilepsies and teaching others about epilepsy. We hope that the third edition of this book will be read by everyone involved with epilepsy, including people with epilepsy themselves, by their parents, carers and relatives and by members of the nursing, teaching and social work professions who would like a clear and accurate introduction to this group of disorders.

Richard E. Appleton
Anthony G. Marson

Contents

1

What is epilepsy?

> ## ➲ Key points
>
> ◆ The human brain has over 100,000 million nerve cells.
>
> ◆ Epileptic seizures occur when nerve cells fire abnormally and synchronously.
>
> ◆ Not all seizures are due to epilepsy.
>
> ◆ There are numerous types of seizures.
>
> ◆ There are many potential causes of epilepsy.
>
> ◆ Epilepsy is diagnosed after two or more seizures.
>
> ◆ Epilepsy is common, affecting 3–4 per cent of people by the time they reach the age of 75.
>
> ◆ Epileptic seizures will stop with drug treatment for at least 60 per cent of people.

How nerve cells work

The human brain contains about 100,000 million nerve cells, each of which is connected to many others, perhaps as many as 50,000 others. The brain is the organ of our thinking, memory and emotion. It integrates information from the outside world and so allows us to perceive objects, such as those we can see, hear, touch or smell, and enables us to perceive events around us. It organizes our response to these events by movements or other actions. It organizes our social behaviour.

Messages are passed between nerve cells by the extraordinarily rapid secretion of tiny packets of specialized chemicals known as neurotransmitters. As a neurotransmitter acts on the next cell in a chain, a brief electric current is generated. These can be recorded by very fine wires placed next to or in a nerve cell, but they are not large enough to be recorded externally over the skin of the head. However, some cells act in rhythmic concert, and these rhythms can be detected with devices such as the electroencephalogram (EEG), a test in which electrodes are placed over the scalp and these electrical rhythms are amplified and recorded digitally or on tape or disc, and displayed on a computer screen, or rarely, a moving strip of paper. The use of this procedure is described in Chapter 5.

Some messages received by a nerve cell are inhibitory—they dampen down the activity of the receiving cell. Some are excitatory, enhancing its activity. The receiving nerve cell computes, as it were, these contrasting messages, which determine its own action.

The events leading to a seizure

One of the ways in which events can go wrong is when a nerve cell loses some of its inputs from other cells because of damage to these other nerve cells. If inhibitory terminals are lost, then the cell will become over-excitable, and begin to switch on, or fire inappropriately, driving other nerve cells with which it is connected. This may result in more and more nerve cells being incorporated into the abnormal pattern of firing.

Thus during an epileptic seizure the normal, quiet, and integrated function of nerve cells in the cerebral hemispheres is interrupted. Instead, nerve cells are forced, through the contacts they make with and receive from other nerve cells, into an abnormal firing pattern, and as the seizure develops, more and more nerve cells become involved. These nerve fibres fire synchronously in paroxysms.

There are a number of different types of seizures, and these are a reflection of different patterns of paroxysmal discharge of nerve cells. Seizure types are described in Chapter 2 and two examples are given here. If the seizure discharge spreads throughout large areas of the brain, then consciousness may be lost. If the discharge of nerve cells is confined to one small area, such as to part of the temporal lobe of the brain (more or less above and in front of the ears), the person may remain conscious but experience a distortion of memory so that the person perceives that he or she has experienced ongoing events before - the phenomenon of déjà vu.

The definition of an epileptic seizure

It is difficult to give a short definition of a seizure, due to the different types of seizure that may occur and the range of symptoms that may be experienced by the person having a seizure, and the range of features that may be observed. An epileptic seizure occurs when there is an abnormal paroxysmal discharge of nerve cells in the cerebral cortex that causes symptoms for the person and/or changes apparent to an observer. The precise symptoms and changes will depend on where in the brain the seizure starts where and how far it spreads. For example, a seizure starting in the temporal lobe may start with a sensation of déjà vu. A seizure rapidly spreading to both cerebral hemispheres might have no warning symptoms, but an observer might see the person go stiff and then shake all four limbs (a convulsion).

In someone with established epilepsy, the EEG between seizures may also show abnormal discharges which are not apparent to the doctor in terms of observed behaviour, nor are they associated with any change perceived by the person with epilepsy. Although the abnormal discharges of the EEG are clearly a fragment, as it were, of a seizure, they are not usually regarded as seizures, as no change is noticed by the person or observer.

The definition of epilepsy

Not all seizures are due to epilepsy. For example, some poisons (or drugs) might cause a person to have a seizure, and similarly an alcoholic might have a seizure whilst withdrawing from alcohol. Without the poison or alcohol withdrawal, these individuals would not have seizures, and they would not be said to have epilepsy. A person is said to have epilepsy if they have recurring seizures (more than two) for which no such provoking factor is found.

There are, however, many grey areas which can cause confusion, some of which are discussed later in this book. Take for example the case of a young man who has a single seizure at the age of 19, the day following a late night and heavy alcohol intake. It would be justifiable to assume that alcohol played some part in the cause of the seizure, but there were others who drank just as much who did not have a seizure. So we must presume that the man has a lower seizure threshold than his friends (see Chapter 3).

A single seizure is not considered sufficient to make the diagnosis of epilepsy, and a diagnosis of epilepsy is usually made following two or more seizures. Around one half of people who have a first seizure will go on to have a second one over the next three years.

Again, there may be grey areas in applying this definition of epilepsy to everyone who has had two seizures. Consider a man who had a seizure at the age of 19 and another at the age of 80. It would seem a bit nonsensical to tell the elderly man that he had had epilepsy all his life, as we would be obliged to do if we followed this definition rigidly. Similarly, consider a woman aged 40, who had ten seizures between the ages of 15 and 25. Although her epilepsy might be considered to still be in remission, she remains at a small risk of having a seizure. Should we consider her as someone with epilepsy? These examples hopefully show that the label 'epilepsy' has to be applied with common sense. It is not one of those tidy diseases such as myocardial infarction, in which there is little argument about the heart attack or the coronary disease causing it.

These medical uncertainties and complexities can make it difficult to give a crystal clear definition and explanation of the illness. Epilepsy is a common condition that has been recognized since ancient times, and there is a common folklore around epilepsy which is full of half truths and inaccuracies. Half truths, include the notion that epilepsy always starts in childhood, is inherited, and is always convulsive in nature. Inaccuracies include the notions that epilepsy is a mental illness and that women with epilepsy cannot have children. Some of these half truths and misconceptions can be a cause of major stigma to people with epilepsy. In this book, we hope to provide some clarity about epilepsy and dispel these ideas.

Identifying the cause of epilepsy

Once a doctor has decided that a person has epilepsy, the next question to address is usually, why? There are many, many potential causes of epilepsy, and the doctor will usually have a good idea as to the cause according to the types of seizure and the age of the person. For up to two-thirds of the people, no specific cause is found, and for many of these the cause is thought be genetic; epilepsies with a genetic cause most commonly start in childhood and adolescence. If the doctor thinks that the seizures are unlikely to be genetic in origin, a brain scan—computerized tomography (CT) or magnetic resonance imaging (MRI)—is usually undertaken to try and identify a brain abnormality that is causing the epilepsy. On average, serious causes such as brain tumours are only found in around one in a hundred people.

Words used to describe epileptic seizures

Doctors and patients use many different words to describe seizures. The most readily recognized seizure in which a patient collapses, goes rigid and then had rhythmic shaking of all four limbs might be called a convulsion, a fit, a grand mal attack, a generalized seizure, or a tonic–clonic seizure. The latter, tonic–clonic seizure, is the preferred medical term and will be used throughout this book. The different types of seizures are described in more detail later in this book. Throughout this book we use the word 'seizure' to refer to all seizures types except febrile convulsions, which are described in Chapter 9. In clinical practice, doctors will often use the words used by their patients such as fit, turn, attack or dizzy spell. People who have two types of seizure often call them 'big ones' and 'little ones'. As long as the patient and the doctor find themselves talking about the same events, this is perfectly acceptable.

Sometimes in correspondence and conversation doctors employ the words epileptiform or epileptoid. In our experience, doctors who use such terms are skating round the subject and avoiding frankly stating that their patient has had an epileptic seizure.

How common is epilepsy?

The incidence of a disease is a measure of the number of new cases in a defined population (usually 100,000) in a defined period of time (usually one year).

There have been a number of good research studies that have estimated the incidence of new cases of epilepsy, one of which was a study of the population of Olmstead County in Minnesota. People in this rural part of the USA do not move around very much, and have the good fortune to be cared for by doctors at the famous Mayo Clinic.

Research workers there have long had an interest in identifying all patients with epilepsy. Figure 1.1 shows the incidence of new cases of epilepsy (more than one non-febrile seizure) per 100,000 per year plotted against the age of onset. The incidence of new cases is highest in infancy and in old age for reasons which are explained in Chapter 3, but new cases can occur at any age. Throughout middle life the incidence is about 40 cases per 100,000 per year. As the years go by, the risk of having had epilepsy at some time in one's life increases in a cumulative fashion. From the United States study cited above, the cumulative risk by age 75 was 3,400 per 100,000 (3.4 per cent) for males and 2,800 per 100,000 (2.8 per cent) for females. In other words, anyone reaching the age of 75 has a 3–4 per cent chance of having had a diagnosis of epilepsy. Epilepsy is thus not a rare or unusual disorder; seizures may impinge upon the lives of anyone of us.

Prevalence is another measure used to assess how common a disease is. This is a measure of how many people in the population actually have a disease at

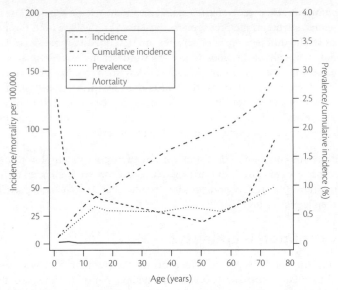

Figure 1.1 Incidence and cumulative incidence, prevalence and mortality rates for epilepsy in the Rochester, Minnesota (1935–1974) study. With permission from Anderson VE, Howser WA, Rich S.

any particular point in time. Prevalance is usually expressed as the number of cases per 1,000 population. Studying prevalence requires methods that are time-consuming and expensive, such as door to door surveys or in-depth study of all potential cases registered with general practitioners. Studying the prevalence of epilepsy is also complicated by a need to decide who should be classified as having ongoing or 'active' epilepsy. The sort of definition used typically is anyone who has had two or more seizures in their life, has had a seizure in the past two years and/or is taking anti-epileptic drug treatment. Estimates of prevalence around the world vary, but typical estimates for the developed world are 0.5 to 1 per cent. In other words, at any one time between 0.5 per cent and 1 per cent of the population have epilepsy. This again indicates that epilepsy is a common condition.

As seen in Figure 1.1 epilepsy may often start in the elderly. In western societies, people are living longer and there are more elderly people than ever before, which obviously means that there will be more elderly people with epilepsy. Recent research has even suggested that as a result of this, in some countries, it is now more common for epilepsy to start in the elderly than in children. However, it must also be emphasized that it is often difficult to diagnose epileptic seizures in the elderly. The elderly are more likely to have multiple medical problems and might have falls or blackouts for a number of reasons and a careful history should be taken to help differentiate epileptic seizures from other events. For example blackouts may occur due to a heart problem, or due to a side-effect of treatment for another condition including hypertension or hypotension. Getting a good and accurate description from an eye-witness is essential, but sometimes made difficulty by the fact that increasing numbers of elderly people live alone following the death of their partner.

Does epilepsy stop?

There is one encouraging point that all those with epilepsy must remember: with anti-epileptic drug treatment, seizures stop for around 60 per cent of people. For the majority, seizures will be controlled in the first 1–2 years after starting treatment although for some there may be a period of attempting to find the right treatment or right combination of treatments before seizures may be controlled. Sometimes, surgery may help put seizures into remission. The chances of success with drugs or surgery depend in part upon the cause of the epilepsy and this is discussed in more detail in Chapter 6. For patients whose seizures have stopped, around half can stop treatment without seizures recurring. However, it is difficult to predict precisely who will have a recurrence and who will not, and many people decide to continue taking treatment rather than risk coming off treatment.

2

The different types of epileptic seizure and epilepsy syndromes

⊃ Key points

- Epilepsy is not a single condition but a group of conditions.

- There are many types of epileptic seizures: these are usually divided into generalized and focal (also called partial) seizures.

- Some types of seizures are easy to identify but others are not, particularly in infants and young children.

- There are many types of epilepsy; these are often referred to as epilepsy syndromes.

- Most epilepsy syndromes occur in children.

- Identifying and diagnosing an epilepsy syndrome may provide useful information on the likely outcome of the epilepsy and how to treat it.

Strictly speaking the term 'epilepsy' should be replaced by the term 'epilepsies', because there are so many different types of epilepsy. This is also true for epileptic seizures—of which there are many different types. Figure 2.1 illustrates the two main types or classes of origin of seizure—focal (also called partial) and generalized. In the top part of the figure, the coloured area indicates a number of nerve cells in the cortex (the name given to the layers of nerve cells on the surface of the brain) which are in some way abnormal, tending to discharge in a sudden or paroxysmal pattern. They may drive other nerve cells to follow their abnormal patterns of discharge. The paths of influence of the discharging nerve cells are indicated by the arrows. As long as the discharge remains in one part of the brain, the seizure is said to be a focal or partial seizure. The older term, 'localization-related', for partial or focal is now no longer used. What happens during a focal seizure depends upon the exact site and pattern of discharge of abnormal nerve cells. Complex partial seizures arising from the temporal lobe are of this type and are described in more detail later on in this chapter, along with those of other types of focal seizures.

The abnormal discharge may spread through the nerve connections linking the two halves of the brain (which is called the corpus callosum), or by affecting poorly identified central collections of cells, initiating a generalized seizure discharge, in which case the seizure is said to be a focal or partial seizure with secondary generalization (to a convulsive or tonic–clonic seizure). These are also known as tonic–clonic seizures for reasons which are explained on p. 12. This process is shown in the middle illustration of Fig. 2.1.

The bottom illustration of Fig. 2.1 shows the second main class of seizure. In this class of seizures, central collections of nerve cells are in some way abnormal in their behaviour or function—even though they may appear to be perfectly normal when examined under the microscope. Because of their central position, and the direction and power of their transmissions, a seizure discharge generated within them spreads more or less simultaneously to all parts of the brain. Because this type of seizure is thought to involve all parts of the brain simultaneously at its onset, it is called a primary generalized seizure. Typical absence (previously known as petit mal) seizures, and some tonic–clonic seizures, are of this type.

It is possible that with future research it may be shown that the differentiation between partial and generalized seizures is not as obvious as it would appear to be at the current time.

Tonic–clonic seizures

Whether the paroxysmal discharge is primary, or secondarily generalized from a focus in the cerebral cortex, consciousness is generally lost if the seizure discharge involves most of the brain and certainly if it involves all of the brain.

Cerebral nerve cells are connected to other nerve cells in the spinal cord. The powerful generalized cortical seizure discharge is therefore linked through this direct transmission system to muscle fibres. Disordered contraction of all muscles is the hallmark of a tonic–clonic seizure.

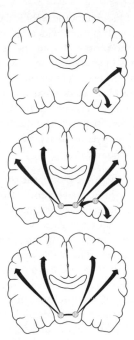

Figure 2.1 Different types of epileptic seizure. *Top:* Focal or partial seizure–the paroxysmal discharge spreads locally from a focus of abnormal cells in the cortex, here folded in within the temporal lobe. *Middle:* Focal or partial seizure with secondary generalization–the discharge spreads locally, and also to centrally grouped nerve cells which spread the discharge widely through the brain. *Bottom:* Primary generalized seizure–the discharge spreads symmetrically throughout the brain from its start or onset.

The first phase of a tonic–clonic seizure is known as the tonic (contraction) phase. At this stage, because of widespread contraction of muscles, the body is rigid, and is incapable of maintaining a normal coordinated posture, so the person falls to the ground. The respiratory muscles also contract, forcing out the air from the chest, so there may be an involuntary noise—a grunt or a cry—at the onset of the tonic phase of the seizure. The jaw muscles also contract, and because the normal associated movements that keep the tongue out of the way are disordered by the seizure discharge, the tongue or the inside of the cheek may be bitten, resulting in blood appearing in the saliva or on the pillow, or both. During the tonic phase there are no coordinated movements of breathing, yet muscular contraction caused by the seizure discharge is vigorous. This combination means that the oxygen in the blood is rapidly used up, and the person will become a dusky blue colour, the technical name for which is cyanosis. This colour is exaggerated by dilatation (widening) of blood vessels in the face by raised pressure within the thorax, due to the strong contraction of chest muscles. Normal movements of swallowing are lost, so that saliva may dribble out between the tightly clenched teeth. The disordered contraction of abdominal and bladder muscles may result in incontinence of urine, though this is by no means invariable. Rarely there may also be disordered contraction of the rectum which may result in some faecal incontinence; this occurs much less commonly than urinary incontinence. The eyes are usually open and dilatation (widening) of the pupils and sweating often occur.

After one or two minutes of the tonic phase, the seizure passes into the clonic (convulsive) phase, with rhythmic movements of the limbs and trunk muscles. The movements in the clonic phase gradually increase in frequency over 30–60 seconds and then gradually decrease over another one or two minutes. As the clonic phase comes to a stop, the rhythmic jerking movements become slightly stronger but less frequent. The whole tonic–clonic seizure usually lasts three to five minutes. After the seizure has finished, the child or adult lies passively unconscious, often breathing very noisily. Normal colour then returns, usually quite quickly. Consciousness gradually lightens, so that the individual can be roused, begin to move around, and then can be helped to their feet and sit in a chair. For several minutes after this, they will be confused and restless. After this, they may have quite a bad headache for the rest of the day, or they may go to bed and sleep for up to two or three hours, occasionally longer. They will also be aware of stiff and painful muscles which have contracted forcibly during the seizure. The following day many people will feel washed-out and have little or no energy and appetite.

Typical absence (previously called petit mal) seizures

Although a translation of 'petit mal' is the 'little illness', petit mal does not mean the same as 'minor epilepsy' as there are all sorts of small attacks which are not attacks of petit mal. The term petit mal should no longer be used as the term confuses people—including doctors who have a limited understanding about epilepsy. True absence (petit mal) seizures are, by definition, associated with a characteristic EEG discharge, illustrated in Chapter 5. Short-lived focal or partial seizures arising from a focus of abnormal nerve cells in one temporal lobe of the brain may be a little similar on clinical grounds, but the distinction is important to make because of the differences in cause, treatment, and outcome between these two types of seizure.

Absence epilepsy is nearly always a disorder of childhood and hardly ever starts in adults. A typical absence seizure is described as follows:

- it occurs very suddenly, like a switch being turned off

- the child will suddenly stop, often in the middle of what they are doing or saying, stare, develop a glazed, 'far-away' look, possibly flicker their eyelids, lick their lips and even fidget with their hands. Rarely, their head may drop very slightly forwards. The posture of the limbs and trunk is usually maintained so they do not fall

- it is very brief, usually lasting only five to ten seconds, occasionally as long as twenty seconds

- the seizure will end as rapidly as it started

- after the seizure, the child may appear slightly confused for just one or two seconds but then resumes what they were doing before the seizure.

Because the interruption of the normal stream of consciousness is so brief, attacks may be unobserved by parents, and not commented on by the child themselves. However, after a seizure the child may be aware that something has happened—but not exactly what. Sometimes, it is the child's teacher who first recognizes the child apparently 'switching off' in class and will suggest that the child is taken to their general practitioner, to see whether they might have petit mal epilepsy. One of us has seen a typical absence seizure in a supermarket. A girl aged about six was in a shop buying a toy and was about to give the money to the shop assistant. She suddenly paused with her hand held outstretched, flickered her eyes for four or five seconds, and then continued handing over the money to the assistant. It is very important to understand that absence seizures typically interrupt or temporarily stop activities and conversation, unlike simple daydreams (which are far more common in children), which do not interrupt activities and usually occur when the child is bored and watching television.

Whereas it is very uncommon to have more than one tonic–clonic seizure in a day, absence seizures may be very frequent—occurring 20 or even 50 (or many more) times per day, every day. Fortunately most children with absence seizures will only be seen to have 10 or 20 seizures each day.

Both tonic–clonic and absence seizures are often characterized by bodily jerks, called myoclonic seizures, which are particularly frequent soon after waking—after either a night's sleep or daytime nap. These are brief, shock-like contractions of the muscles, which are so short-lived that they be missed by those observing the person having them. One or both arms or legs or the whole body may be involved. This is often called the 'flying saucer syndrome' in reference to the broken plates or saucers that may result from these myoclonic seizures happening at breakfast time. Affected children are often described as 'butter-fingers' or 'clumsy' because of these jerks—which may have been happening for many months or years, without being diagnosed as being a type of epileptic seizure.

Focal—also called partial—seizures

The exact internal perception or external appearance of focal or partial seizures depends upon the site of origin of discharge of abnormal nerve cells, that is, exactly where the seizure is starting from in the brain. If these lie in the part of the brain called the motor cortex, a strip of brain concerned with movement (Figure 2.2), the initial manifestation will be a contraction of muscles on the opposite side of the body, as one side of the brain controls the opposite side of the body. Brain cells (neurons) in the motor cortex which supply the index finger and thumb, the corner of the mouth, or the big toe are most likely to be those in which a seizure discharge begins. There are more nerve cells assigned to controlling these muscles, which are concerned with the fine-tuning of manual skills and facial expressions. Statistically, therefore, there is a greater chance of abnormal events occurring in these nerve cells; experiments also show that they are particularly easy to excite. The first evidence of such a focal or partial seizure may be twitching of one corner of the mouth.

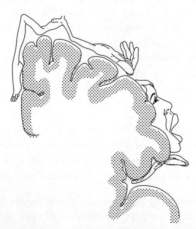

Figure 2.2 A section of the brain (same orientation as in Figure 2.1), showing the motor cortex and a drawing of the parts of the body controlled by different areas (after Penfield).

As the seizure discharge spreads, the muscles in the face and particularly around the eyes are next involved, as nerve cells serving these muscles are located next to those serving the mouth. Next involved are the hand muscles, and the seizure may then travel up the arm and then start to affect the foot and leg muscles. This march of events was described in the last century, independently by Bravais, a French neurologist, and by Hughlings Jackson, an English neurologist whose wife had such attacks. This type of seizure is therefore often called a Jacksonian seizure. The site of origin of this focal seizure is usually within one of the frontal lobes. It generally occurs with no disturbance of consciousness, as the discharge remains confined to the motor cortex. Seizures in which there is no disturbance of consciousness used to be called 'simple partial seizures', but now such a seizure would be described as a focal seizure, followed by a very detailed description of what exactly happened during the seizure.

Another type of focal seizure with movement is known as a versive (turning) seizure. In this the head and eyes turn to one side.

Usually the arm on the side to which they are turned is elevated and twisted: the medical term for which is dystonia and it may also twitch or jerk. Sometimes the version may continue so that the subject turns round and round several times. Version is usually in the direction away from the discharging cerebral nerve cells—whereby a focus of abnormal nerve cells in the left hemisphere causes turning to the right. Such seizures are therefore called adversive. This type of focal seizure also usually arises from one of the frontal lobes.

In the types of focal seizures described so far, there is an external manifestation—a contraction of muscles driven by the discharging cerebral nerve cells—so that this type of seizure is easily apparent to an observer.

However, other groups of discharging cerebral nerve cells may not necessarily result in any apparent external event, only in a distorted internal perception, or abnormal sensation which is felt by the person having the seizure. These are usually called auras, but are still a type of simple partial or focal seizure, although rather subtle. The precise type or description of the sensory seizure will depend upon where it is coming from. These can include the following:

- a seizure coming from a focus in one parietal lobe (situated just behind the motor cortex) may only result in a transient disturbance of sensation, such as a perception of pins and needles, numbness or heaviness in the opposite side of the face, arm, or leg.

◆ a seizure discharge in the anterior part of one temporal lobe may result only in the person perceiving a strange smell, unreal, often unpleasant, and yet often vaguely familiar. Similar hallucinations of distorted taste may also occur, which are usually perceived as unpleasant. Sometimes the sensation is one of sudden and very unpleasant fear which can result in the person screaming for no obvious reason and not being able to be comforted.

◆ if the seizure discharge begins in a slightly different part of the temporal lobe—the posterior temporal lobe—complex visual hallucinations may occur. A boy of 11 told one of us that he saw himself standing near a shower with another boy, whom he felt he knew but could not name. This boy and he alternately put their feet under the running water, and this odd hallucination continued until the seizure ended, after which the child felt very sleepy.

◆ other seizures arising in the temporal lobe may cause a perception that events taking place have previously occurred in precisely the same way in the person's experience. This phenomenon is known as déjà vu. 'Jamais vu' is a phrase used to indicate that the person perceives familiar surroundings as being completely unreal.

◆ a seizure that originates from the occipital lobe (the part of the brain at the back of the head) may cause the person to have visual hallucinations but these are often much simpler than the hallucinations that come from the posterior part of the temporal lobe. Occipital lobe hallucinations usually consist of multicoloured spots, lines or geometric shapes rather than bizarre pictures.

If such distorted perceptions occur they may disturb full consciousness—as defined by awareness of current events, interpretation of current events, and correct responsiveness to current events. All degrees of disturbance of consciousness may be seen. For example, the child or adult may respond appropriately to a question after a considerable delay, or they may respond inappropriately, or not at all. After the attack has terminated, people may say that they were partly aware of ongoing real events, but this is not necessarily true, and the person may have no memory for all events during and for some time after the seizure. Partial seizures in which consciousness is disturbed used to be called complex partial seizures. Now they are described as a focal seizure followed by a very detailed, second-by-second description, of what exactly happens during the seizure.

Sometimes seizures arising in the temporal lobe result in complex automatic behaviour—a so-called psychomotor seizure. The person may, for example, dress and undress repeatedly or drum their fingers on the table. Less complex, but common manifestations, includes repeated sucking or chewing or swallowing movements. The person will have no memory for these events after the attack.

Such automatic behaviour occurring during the seizure discharge must be distinguished from the common confusion following a tonic–clonic seizure, or following a prolonged temporal lobe seizure, for which the person will also be amnesic, meaning a loss of memory. This amnesia is, perhaps, very similar to the amnesia following a head injury, in which, for example, a young man will complete a game of rugby football after a collision resulting in a concussive head injury, yet afterwards he will be amnesic for this part of the game, and have no recollection of the head injury.

Emotional experiences are very frequent in partial seizures arising in the temporal lobe. These are often expressed just as 'a horrible feeling', but sometimes the sensation of fear or panic is overpowering.

Sensations in the abdomen and chest often also occur. A common initial sensation is a vague feeling of discomfort in the upper abdomen, which rises rapidly into the chest and head. The abdominal sensation may be accompanied by contractions of the stomach and bowel resulting in audible rumbles; children may sometimes describe this feeling like having 'butterflies in the tummy' or as if 'I am going to be sick'.

A less frequent internal sensation is one of vertigo. People with seizures beginning in the temporal lobe may say that they are 'dizzy'. This word is used in different senses by various people, but some appear to perceive vertigo (a sense of disequilibrium which may be rotational, which means that the room appears to be spinning or the person feels that they are falling to one side) as part of the seizure.

Most people are right-handed, the left hemisphere then being considered to be dominant. Language is very largely located in the dominant hemisphere. An aphasic focal seizure in which expression (speaking) or comprehension (understanding) of language is impaired may arise from a seizure discharge in the dominant temporal lobe. In addition, when someone is unable to speak for many minutes after a focal or partial seizure, it suggests that the seizure has originated from the person's dominant temporal lobe, which is usually the left temporal lobe.

Any focal seizure (the types previously called simple or complex partial seizures), may become secondarily generalized into a tonic–clonic seizure (see Figure 2.1). Sometimes this happens so quickly that not even someone who is there at the start of the seizure will notice that it has a focal onset. The fact that it *starts* as a focal or partial seizure will only become apparent on careful analysis of an EEG recorded at the time of the seizure itself.

Rarer types of seizure

Atypical absences (previously called a petit mal variant)

This phrase is used in two different ways—to describe absences which are clinically similar to typical absences associated with an EEG record that is not typical and also to describe absences in association with other clinical features which are not typical. These clinical features include loss of postural control of the head or body or repeated jerks (myoclonic seizures) affecting the eyes, head or limbs. These seizures may be called myoclonic absences, eyelid myoclonia with absences or myoclonic-astatic seizures. Some of these epilepsies may cause the individual (most commonly a child) to crash or 'drop' to the floor with such force and frequency that they have to wear a crash helmet to protect their head from damage. Sometimes the myoclonic–astatic seizures are called drop seizures. Other types of seizures may also result in what appear to be drop seizures and these are called atonic (meaning loss of tone or posture—like a puppet's strings being suddenly cut) and tonic (meaning that the person suddenly stiffens and may fall, like a tree being felled).

Clonic seizures

The distinction between these and myoclonic jerks is slight. If jerks are multiple and repeated very quickly, then the seizures tend to be called clonic.

Tonic seizures

A tonic (rigid) posturing of all limbs without a clonic phase is sometimes seen in some generalized brain disorders in childhood. Tonic seizures are unpleasant seizures as the person will suddenly fall—rather like a tree being felled. Tonic seizures are very commonly seen in a severe type of epilepsy syndrome called the Lennox-Gastaut syndrome (named after two famous doctors specializing in epilepsy in the 1950s). The name Lennox-Gastaut is given to one very rare form of focal seizure in which one part of the body briefly maintains abnormal tonic posture. Such seizures may occasionally occur in adults with multiple sclerosis. It is thought that this type of focal seizure may start from one of the frontal lobes.

Infantile spasms (salaam seizures; West syndrome)

These seizures occur in infancy and typically start between 3 and 12 months of age. The most likely age at which they start is between 6 and 9 months of age. They are characterized by a brief, sudden flexion of head, trunk, and limbs, as if the baby is bowing a 'salaam'. The infant may appear to be thrown forwards or backwards with the arms outstretched. Each spasm lasts about one, or at most two, seconds. The spasms may occur in runs or clusters (from five to up to fifty spasms per cluster) over a 5–15 minute period; when this happens the infant may appear distressed afterwards and cry. If the spasms have been occurring for some weeks or months, the child's development can appear to come to a stop or the child may even lose some skills. Their sleep pattern becomes disturbed. Sometimes these infants can appear to have problems seeing and can even be thought to have become blind. Spasms are more likely to occur at certain times of the day, particularly just after the infant has woken up from a sleep, or is about to fall asleep. In some children, the spasms may occur almost continuously throughout the day, happening several times an hour. The EEG in infants with this type of seizure shows very abnormal patterns of activity called hypsarrhythmia (Chapter 5). When the spasms are controlled with medication and the EEG improves then the child's development may also start to improve, although this is not always the case because the outcome will also depend on the cause of the infantile spasms.

Doctors also now recognize that spasms may occur in older children, and these are then called epileptic spasms. This type of seizure is also thought to come from one of the frontal lobes and is usually easier to treat than infantile spasms.

The frequency with which different types of seizure occur

The best information about this comes from studies carried out in general practice (Table 2.1). However, it must be emphasized that these figures are likely to be only approximate at best because of difficulties in the correct diagnosis of both epilepsy and the specific type of epileptic seizure. Tonic– clonic seizures and infantile/epileptic spasms are not included in this table because it is often difficult to recognize these seizures, particularly in young children.

Table 2.1 Proportion in percentages of the type of seizure six months after onset of epilepsy in 564 people (all ages) (data from the National General Practice Study of Epilepsy)

Seizure type	%
Classifiable	91.0
Unclassifiable	9.0
Generalized seizures	39.0
Tonic–clonic	35.0
Absences	1.0
Myoclonic	<1.0
Other generalized types	2.5
Partial (focal) seizures	53.0
Simple	3.0
Complex	11.0
Partial evolving to secondarily generalized	27.0

Further definitions

There are a few more aspects of epileptic seizures that require explanation.

Prodrome

Some people may have a warning of a seizure. The first type of warning is a vague feeling of an impending seizure, particularly before a tonic–clonic seizure. This prodrome may last several hours. It has no obvious physiological explanation, but it is remarked upon too often by people to be completely dismissed as being due to an imaginary reconstruction of events. The prodrome is usually unpleasant—a feeling of mental heaviness or depression. Less commonly, elation and energetic activity may herald a seizure. Parents of children and relatives may notice a change in a person's behaviour—with them becoming very restless, moody or bad-tempered—for many minutes, hours, or, rarely, days before a seizure.

Aura

The second type of warning, known as an aura, is not really a warning at all, but the initial symptom of the seizure itself. An aura is actually an example of what used to be called a simple partial seizure. Examples of such auras include the epigastric sensation (a feeling that seems to come from the stomach) of a focal seizure arising in one part of the temporal lobe, or the brief tingling in one hand which precedes a focal seizure arising in the parietal lobe, or coloured shapes and circles which precede a focal seizure arising in the occipital lobe. All of these auras may then become secondarily generalized, progressing into a tonic–clonic seizure.

Post-ictal paresis

An ictus is another, older name for a seizure. Post-ictal paresis indicates weakness of the left or right side of the body following a tonic–clonic convulsion primarily affecting those limbs. Sometimes known as Todd's paresis, after the name of the neurologist who first described it, it usually indicates some structural abnormality or problem in the hemisphere on the side opposite to the weak limbs. However, a structural cause is not always found, even with very detailed brain scans. The weakness may last from a few minutes up to 48 hours.

Post-ictal amnesia, post-ictal confusion, post-ictal sleep, and post-ictal headache have already been described. Post-ictal automatism is the phenomenon in which a person can undertake some fairly complex behaviours or acts, such as undressing and putting themselves to bed, of which they have no subsequent memory.

Status epilepticus

Status epilepticus is a phrase used to indicate seizures occurring so close together that one seizure runs into another, without recovery of normal cerebral function between seizures. This may happen with any type of seizure, so that status can be divided up into:

◆ absence status (which could be typical or atypical)

◆ focal (complex partial) status

◆ tonic–clonic (convulsive) status.

In the first two types, which are often collectively called 'non-convulsive' or 'electrical' status epilepticus, a diagnosis that may be very difficult to reach. The person may be found in the street or at home, confused and inaccessible to conversation because of continuing seizure discharges. Non-convulsive status epilepticus is more likely to occur in individuals with a more severe type of epilepsy such as Lennox–Gastaut syndrome, severe myoclonic epilepsy of infancy and myoclonic-astatic epilepsy and is therefore more commonly seen in children. Doctors should always listen to parents of children with epilepsy when they say that their child is 'not quite right', or 'there is something wrong with him—he can't speak or eat properly' or 'he is dribbling all the time'— because the child may be in non-convulsive status epilepticus. The diagnosis may be easily confirmed, or excluded, by doing an EEG during the period of changed or confused behaviour. This is why non-convulsive status epilepticus is also known as electrical status epilepticus. Non-convulsive status epilepticus occurs repeatedly in individuals with the more severe epilepsies and may be very hard to treat. However, it is not usually a medical emergency and people can be in non-convulsive status epilepticus for days or weeks and when it ceases, the person is usually back to normal within minutes.

Convulsive or tonic–clonic status epilepticus, in which the person does not recover consciousness between generalized tonic–clonic convulsions, is, however, a medical emergency. The lack of normal breathing, together with the extreme muscular contractions during the seizure, throws a considerable stress upon the heart and the cardiovascular system as well as on the brain. If the episode of tonic–clonic status lasts for more than 60 minutes without stopping, then the person's brain may suffer irreversible damage and the person may even die. This is because the brain is deprived of oxygen and glucose (energy) and as a result, it swells and this in turn causes the death of nerve cells. The principles of treatment of this serious but fortunately uncommon state are discussed in Chapter 6, but early treatment and admission to hospital are essential.

Epilepsia partialis continua

Finally, a focal seizure in which the seizure discharge continues but remains confined to one part of the motor cortex (resulting in continuous twitching of muscles in one part of a limb on the opposite side of the body) is called epilepsia partialis continua. For example, the index finger and thumb may continue to twitch for days or even weeks, without any spread of seizure discharge to other muscles, and with no disturbance of consciousness. It is also called the Kojewnikov syndrome after the neurologist who first described it. This is a very rare but severe form of focal status and is usually caused by a structural, metabolic or infectious disorder that affects the brain. Two of these disorders are Rasmussen's syndrome (previously called Rasmussen's encephalitis) and mitochondrial disorder. Viral encephalitis such as that caused by herpes simplex may also cause epilepsia partialis continua. All of these disorders are usually associated with a poor outcome, with the person continuing to experience very frequent seizures and also developing a severe weakness down the affected side of the body.

Epilepsy syndromes

The first part of this chapter discussed most of the different types of epileptic seizures. Paediatricians and neurologists recognize that certain clusters of symptoms, signs, and patients' characteristics go together to produce a recognizable pattern, and this is what is meant by a syndrome. The concept—or suggestion—of epilepsy syndromes goes back many years, but a revised scheme or classification of epilepsy was proposed by the International League Against Epilepsy (ILAE) in 1989. The new classification proposed by the ILAE in 2001 includes a few more epilepsy syndromes than were mentioned in the 1989 classification. In this classification, an epileptic syndrome is characterized by both clinical and EEG findings. On the clinical side, this includes:

- the age at which the seizures started

- the type of seizure or seizures if the child has more than one type of seizure

- the family history of epilepsy (if there is one)

- the child's development and neurological findings.

The EEG is also very important, together with the clinical features described above, in helping to identify a particular epilepsy syndrome and this includes its appearance:

- during a seizure (called the ictal EEG)

- between seizures (called the inter-ictal EEG).

Identifying or diagnosing an epilepsy syndrome allows greater precision of diagnosis and helps to decide which may be the most effective anti-epileptic drug. It also provides more useful information on the prognosis of a person's epilepsy than simply classifying seizure types. Prognosis means that the doctor will be able to give more information about whether:

- a cause for the epilepsy is likely to be found

- the person's epilepsy is likely to be easily controlled with anti-epileptic drugs

- the person's epilepsy is likely to ever go away spontaneously (the technical word for this is remission, which is discussed in more detail in Chapter 7)

- the person is likely to have addition problems such as learning difficulties

◆ there is a high or low risk of this epilepsy syndrome happening again in the same family, for instance if the person is a child and their parents are thinking of having another child.

The same type of seizure can occur in different epilepsy syndromes. For example, tonic–clonic seizures can occur in association with typical absences (primary generalized epilepsy in Figure 2.3) or in association with focal seizures (focal epilepsy). Conversely, a person with one syndrome may have seizures of more than one type. For example, a child with idiopathic generalized epilepsy may have both absence and tonic–clonic seizures and may also have myoclonic seizures. A specific example is juvenile myoclonic epilepsy. All (100 per cent of) individuals who develop this epilepsy syndrome will have myoclonic seizures, 60 per cent will have at least one tonic–clonic seizure and 30 per cent will have absence seizures. Another example is children with juvenile-onset absence epilepsy; all of them will have absence seizures and over 30 per cent will also have tonic–clonic seizures.

The 'causes' of these syndromes, insofar as they are known, are considered in Chapter 3.

However, it must be understood that even if an epilepsy syndrome is identified, this does not necessarily give any information about the underlying cause of the epilepsy. Indeed, one example, West syndrome, may have at least 50 different identified causes—and even more may be discovered in the future! In contrast, severe myoclonic epilepsy of infancy (Dravet syndrome) appears to be associated with a few genetic abnormalities, called *mutations*.

Many of the different epilepsy syndromes begin in childhood, and are best characterized by the age at onset (Table 2.2). However, it is still useful and even important to think in terms of the two main divisions of generalized epilepsy, in which the seizure discharge is generalized from the beginning, and focal (partial) epilepsy, in which the seizure begins in one particular focus (part) of the cortex, even if the seizure then becomes a secondary generalized one. Focal or partial epilepsy usually implies some local structural damage to, or disorder of, nerve cells. Two examples would be epilepsy that develops after a severe head injury or after a cerebral (brain) abscess. Other examples are given in Chapter 3.

Some syndromes have common features and a predictable outcome. For example, some children develop focal seizures that particularly occur at night, and are characterized by large EEG spikes over the central and temporal regions of the brain on one side, called the 'rolandic' area of the brain. Others are rather loose collections of a few common characteristics irregularly linked together.

In the opinion of most experts, a particular epilepsy syndrome will only be identified or diagnosed in 60–70 per cent of children with epilepsy. When a particular epilepsy syndrome cannot be identified, then the child's epilepsy must be classified according to the seizure type or types that the child is experiencing. It is then the seizure type or types that are used to give information on the individual's prognosis and which anti-epileptic drug should be prescribed.

The question of inheritance of epilepsy is considered in Chapter 3, but with the almost daily advances in genetic research, the classification of epilepsy syndromes may eventually become replaced by specific epilepsy disorders or

Table 2.2 The more common epilepsy syndromes classified by age of onset

Newborn period	Benign familial neonatal convulsions
	Vitamin B6 (pyridoxine or pyridoxamine defiency/dependency)
Infancy 1–12 months	Ohtahara syndrome (myoclonic and brief tonic seizures)
	Migrating partial seizures in infancy
	West syndrome (Chapters 2 and 6)
Early childhood (1–5 years)	Febrile seizures (Chapter 9)
	Benign myoclonic epilepsy of infancy
	Severe myoclonic epilepsy of infancy (sometimes called Dravet syndrome)
	Early-onset benign partial epilepsy with occipital spikes/paroxysms (also called Panayiotopoulos syndrome)
Later childhood (5–12 years)	Landau–Kleffner syndrome
	Lennox–Gastaut syndrome
	Childhood-onset absence epilepsy
	Myoclonic–astatic epilepsy
	Benign partial epilepsy with centro-temporal spikes (also called benign rolandic epilepsy)
	Benign partial epilepsy with occipital spikes/paroxysms (also called Gastaut syndrome)
Adolescence (>12 years)	Juvenile-onset absence epilepsy
	Juvenile myoclonic epilepsy
	Epilepsy with tonic–clonic seizures on awakening

genetic diseases. However, for the time being, the concept of epilepsy syndromes is helpful and is still being used by doctors who specialize in epilepsy.

The relationship between types of seizure and types of epilepsy

Figure 2.3 shows three interlocking circles, the area of which is roughly proportional to the frequency of occurrence of various types of seizure. The central circle represents tonic–clonic seizures. The left-hand circle represents focal seizures, many of which become secondarily generalized, as indicated by the considerable overlap between the two circles. Most focal seizures arise from some focal area of structural abnormality within the brain, although it is not always easy to find this abnormality, even with detailed brain scans. These seizures can be said to be symptomatic of some underlying problem, and therefore, affected individuals are described as having *symptomatic* epilepsy.

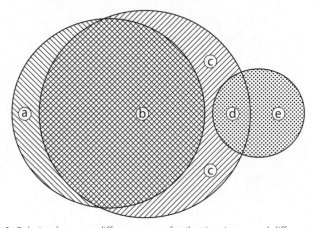

Figure 2.3 Relation between different types of epileptic seizures and different types of epilepsy. a, focal seizures alone; b, focal seizures evolving to tonic–clonic seizures; c, tonic–clonic seizures of uncertain origin; d, tonic–clonic seizures in association with typical absences; e, typical absences alone. a+b, symptomatic epilepsy; c, cryptogenic epilepsy; d+e, idiopathic epilepsy (primary generalized epilepsy).

The right-hand circle represents absence seizures. Between 20–30 per cent of children with absence seizures will also have tonic–clonic seizures, as is indicated by the overlap between right hand and centre circles. The precise percentage of children with absence seizures who will also have tonic–clonic seizures will depend on the specific epilepsy syndrome. Such primary generalized epilepsy is not symptomatic of any underlying structural brain disease, and may be said to be idiopathic epilepsy (the word idiopathic is the technical word meaning 'not known'). It is very likely that many, if not most of the idiopathic epilepsies will be genetically determined.

The area of the centre circle that is not overlapped by the left- and right- hand circles contains those patients who only have tonic–clonic seizures. This group used to be called *cryptogenic* (the word cryptogenic originates from the Greek word, *cryptos*, meaning hidden, as in a 'cryptic' crossword).

The word cryptogenic is no longer used in the ILAE classification, proposed in 2001. It is replaced by 'presumed symptomatic' which means that there must be a cause for the person's epilepsy—but that it hasn't been found yet! It is likely that in the years ahead, with future advances in genetic understanding and more sophisticated EEGs and brain scans, most types of epilepsy and epilepsy syndromes will be found to be either symptomatic or idiopathic.

3

The causes of epilepsy

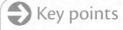 Key points

- There are many causes of epilepsy.

- Doctors must always consider a cause for a person's epilepsy—even though a cause will not always be found.

- A cause will be found in about one third of children with epilepsy.

- A cause will be found in about one half of all people whose epilepsy starts in adult life.

- Brain tumours are a rare cause of epilepsy in children.

- Many people's epilepsy will have a genetic cause—although this does not mean that a definite genetic abnormality will be found.

- Most causes will not be curable or even treatable, although the epilepsy will be treatable.

Once a doctor has made a diagnosis of seizures or epilepsy, the next question to address is what has caused the epilepsy or seizures. To try and identify the cause, the doctor will enquire about past life events that may have caused any brain injury, or any brain insult that may be the cause of the epilepsy such as a severe head injury or meningitis, and ask about other current symptoms which may suggest a particular type of brain-related problem [pathology]. They will also examine the patient, again looking for evidence of brain pathology, and may organise investigations including brain scans (a magnetic resonance imaging [MRI] or computerized tomography [CT] scan) or some blood tests. However, it is important to understand that for many people, a specific cause for their epilepsy or seizures is not found.

When searching for the cause, it is important not to jump to conclusions. For example, minor head injuries are common, and by coincidence a child may have a seizure during the few weeks following a minor head injury. Seizures are in fact rare following minor head injuries, being more common following severe head injuries where the skull has been fractured, and the person has been knocked out for a significant length of time, particularly if a CT or MRI brain scan shows evidence of brain damage caused by the injury.

The same arguments apply when assessing the effects of a difficult birth and the possible relationship of that to the subsequent development of epilepsy. There is no doubt that a very difficult labour, especially if the baby is small, may cause significant brain damage, severe learning difficulties, cerebral palsy, and epilepsy. However, after most difficult or prolonged labours the child develops perfectly and without epilepsy. It is now known that in many children born with cerebral palsy or severe learning difficulties, the problem was not caused by a difficult labour or birth, but that the brain problems occurred before birth. This can include:

- infections passed from the mother to the child during pregnancy (called intrauterine infections)

- abnormal development of the baby's brain (this is usually early on in pregnancy, within the first four months of the pregnancy); this is known as cortical dysplasia and is discussed in more detail later in this chapter

- a problem with the blood and therefore oxygen supply to the baby's brain in the last few days or weeks of pregnancy

Some of the common causes for epilepsy are shown in Table 3.1, and it can be seen that there are different causes at different ages. For example, a structural congenital brain abnormality may cause seizures in young children; head injury is a more common cause in young men; and stroke and degenerative diseases are more common in the elderly. Almost any disease or injury that causes damage in the cerebral cortex can cause epilepsy, and therefore there are potentially thousands of causes of epilepsy. In this chapter, we describe most of the important causes of epilepsy, but we have not attempted to mention or discuss every cause.

Not surprisingly, the causes of epilepsy in the elderly are very different to the causes of epilepsy in children, the other time of life when epilepsy is likely to start. Stroke is the most common cause of damage to the brain in the elderly and occurs either when the blood supply to a part of the brain is blocked (usually by blood clot forming in an artery), or less commonly by a haemorrhage

Causes of epilepsy at different ages

Cause	Newborn	Infant	Child	Adult
Genetic			Idiopathic →	
	-----	Lipidoses -----	→	
	-----	Tuberous sclerosis -----	→	
			Neurofibromatosis →	
			Angioma →	
Congenital	At birth →			
Anoxia*		Febrile convulsions →		
	At birth →			Stroke →
Trauma	At birth →		Head injury →	Head injury →
			Intracranial surgery →	Intercranial surgery →
Tumours			Tumours →	Tumours →
Infectious diseases (bacteria, viruses, parasites)	Meningitis →	Meningitis →	Meningitis →	Meningitis →
		Encephalitis →	Encephalitis →	Encephalitis →
			Abscess →	Abscess →
Acquired metabolic disease	Hypoglycaemia			Chronic renal failure →
	Hypocalcaemia			
Alcohol				Chronic alcohol abuse →
Degenerative disorders				Dementia →

*Reduction of oxygen supply to the brain

(blood leaking into the brain from an artery). A stroke will most commonly cause weakness down one side of the body. The part of the brain that has been damaged by a stroke can then act as a focus for epileptic seizures. Most elderly people starting with epilepsy have not had a stroke, but when investigated, the only abnormality found on a brain scan is signs of damage to the blood supply to the brain, especially if the person has high blood pressure or has been a smoker. At present, more research is needed to identify whether this damage is definitely a cause of epilepsy. Other causes of epilepsy in the elderly include degenerative diseases including Alzheimer's disease, and brain tumours, which could be primary brain tumours (grown from abnormal brain cells), or more likely, secondary tumours that have spread from cancer in other parts of the body such as a lung, breast or the prostate.

Genetic causes of epilepsy

The contribution that genetics makes to the causes of epilepsy remains poorly understood, but there have been major advances in our knowledge over the past 10–15 years. Specific genetic abnormalities have been found for some rare types of epilepsy that tend to run in families (for example a syndrome called Generalized Epilepsy with Febrile Seizures Plus or GEFS+), whilst specific genetic abnormalities have not been found that account for the more common types of epilepsy.

The following types of epilepsy are thought to be purely genetic in origin:

- the idiopathic generalized epilepsies

  - childhood absence epilepsy

  - juvenile absence epilepsy

  - juvenile myoclonic epilepsy

  - epilepsy with tonic–clonic seizures on awaking

- the idiopathic partial epilepsies

  - benign partial epilepsy with centro-temporal spikes

  - benign occipital lobe epilepsy

- other examples of genetic epilepsies

  - severe myoclonic epilepsy of infancy

♦ familial temporal lobe epilepsy with auditory features

♦ autosomal dominant nocturnal frontal lobe epilepsy

These types of epilepsy will usually have specific EEG abnormalities, particularly the idiopathic generalized epilepsies. Whilst these types of epilepsy are thought to be genetic in origin, most people with epilepsy do not have a family member with epilepsy, including those that are thought to have a genetic cause. The precise reason for this is not known. One possible reason is that other family members have the abnormal gene, but only a small number of people with the abnormal gene develop epilepsy (the gene is said to have low penetrance). Another possibility is that a combination of two or more genes is required to cause the epilepsy, so only individuals with a specific combination of abnormal genes develop epilepsy.

There are also a number of rare genetic conditions in which the individual has epilepsy as well as a number of other problems. For example, tuberous sclerosis and neurofibromatosis are rare genetic diseases which cause abnormalities in the brain which can result in epilepsy as well as abnormalities in the skin and other organs. These two conditions are said to have dominant transmission, i.e., each person has two copies of each chromosome and hence two copies of each gene in every cell in their body. Diseases such as tuberous sclerosis and neurofibromatosis occur when the person has one abnormal gene and the other copy of the gene is usually normal. If a person with either of these conditions has a child, there is a 50/50 chance that they will pass on the abnormal gene. Hence, there is a 50/50 chance that the child will also have the condition.

There are other rare genetic diseases in which the gene is said to be recessive, and the individual will develop the disease if both the copies of their gene are abnormal. Parents with one abnormal gene and one normal gene will usually have no symptoms and be unaware that they are carriers of the abnormal gene. If their partner is also a carrier, there is a one in four chance that they will have a child who has two copies of the abnormal gene and will develop the disease. Conditions caused by recessive gene abnormalities are rare, and include disorders of metabolism of the brain, some of which are called lipidoses. Fatty substances known as lipids are important constituents of the membranes surrounding the nerve cells. A disorder of the structure and function of the cell membrane may well lead to paroxysmal discharge of nerve cells—an epileptic seizure. These conditions are associated with epilepsy, significant learning difficulties, impairment of movement and vision and usually with brain degeneration. Fortunately, these conditions are rare.

Other rare genetic conditions which are commonly, if not typically, associated with epilepsy, that is usually hard to treat, include:

◆ Down syndrome (trisomy 21)

◆ Rett syndrome

◆ Angelman syndrome

◆ Miller–Dieker syndrome (due to a major malformation of the brain called lissencephaly or smooth brain)

◆ ring chromosome 20 and 14 syndromes

◆ Alpers syndrome

The genetic contribution to other forms of epilepsy, particularly the focal or partial epilepsies, is more poorly understood. For some people, it is likely that a combination of both a genetic susceptibility and another cause are important. For example, not everyone with a severe head injury or a stroke develops epilepsy. It may be that people with certain genes are more susceptible to developing epilepsy following a head injury or stroke than others. Thus, the head injury or stroke as well as the genetic abnormality are prerequisites to cause the epilepsy. The same may be true for many other causes of brain injury that result in epilepsy. Ongoing research may identify one, or more likely, many genes that are responsible for causing the different types of epilepsy.

Parents and prospective parents with epilepsy will want to know the risk of their own children developing epilepsy; this should be discussed with the doctor who is providing their medical care. Families should be referred for a specialist genetics opinion if the epilepsy is complicated or is accompanied by other medical problems (as in those caused by a metabolic condition).

There are no tests that can be undertaken to predict whether the child will develop epilepsy. The overall risk of developing epilepsy is estimated from knowledge of the parents' family history, the parent's seizure type(s) and the cause of the parent's epilepsy. These risks are:

◆ for the majority of parents with focal onset seizures (simple partial, complex partial and secondary generalized seizures—see page 14) the risk for their children developing epilepsy is only slightly higher than for the general population at around 1 in 20.

◆ for parents with a generalized epilepsy (e.g. absence epilepsy or juvenile myoclonic epilepsy—see pages 10–13), the risk of their child developing epilepsy is higher at around 1 in 10. The risk becomes even higher when one or more of the parents' close relatives also have epilepsy.

Congenital malformations

Some congenital abnormalities (meaning abnormalities of the brain present at birth) are not inherited. For example, the abnormalities in the limbs of the children whose mothers had taken the drug thalidomide during pregnancy are congenital, but will not be passed on to their children, as the thalidomide affected the developing cells in the limbs without causing any mutations in the baby's own ovaries or testes (although there continues to be some debate). Other congenital abnormalities may have an inherited basis.

One congenital abnormality relevant to epilepsy is an abnormal development of blood vessels known as an angioma. The abnormal vessels may be arterial, venous, or capillary. Sometimes a clot or thrombus forms in one or more of the abnormal vessels, exacerbating the situation. One type of capillary angioma of the brain is associated with a similar malformation of blood vessels in the skin of the upper part of the face—the Sturge–Weber syndrome. Children with this particular combination of angiomatous abnormalities have a very high risk of developing epilepsy.

More common than angiomas as a cause of epilepsy are disorders of migration of the nerve cells in the brain during foetal development, so some end up in the wrong place, the wrong layer of the brain, or with the wrong connections with other nerve cells in the brain. This is usually called cortical dysplasia. Cortical dysplasia may affect the whole brain or just one area, when it is called focal cortical dysplasia. There are many different types of cortical dysplasia, some of which are now known to be genetic, but the cause of most cases of cortical dysplasia is still poorly understood. People with cortical dysplasia will most commonly develop epilepsy in early childhood, usually by three to six months of age, and some may develop epilepsy later in life. When the individual has focal cortical dysplasia, they may also have additional problems including:

- hemiparesis (weakness affecting one side of the body)
- visual problems, particularly in the peripheral vision (called the visual fields)
- learning difficulties
- behaviour problems.

Anoxia

Anoxia means lack of sufficient oxygen, an essential component of the normal ongoing chemistry of a cell. Cerebral nerve cells are amongst the highest consumers of oxygen in the body, as reflected in the fact that a quarter of all arterial blood pumped by the heart goes to the brain. If the oxygen supply is cut off for more than a few minutes, then damage to nerve cells may occur. Some nerve cells may die, but others may be damaged in such a way that they may start to function abnormally which can then lead to epilepsy.

Anoxia may occur for many reasons. It may occur at birth:

◆ during each uterine contraction in a prolonged labour the foetal heart rate slows, and the supply of oxygenated blood to the brain is reduced. It may recover between contractions but not always and unless the baby is delivered urgently, they may suffer severe brain damage

◆ the placenta may separate prematurely. As a result, the baby does not receive the blood and therefore, the oxygen they need. This usually causes severe brain damage in the baby

◆ if the child is born prematurely, then they may not breathe properly after birth and the child will again suffer anoxic brain damage

◆ babies that are born very prematurely (before 24 weeks of pregnancy) are also at risk from having a bleed in their brain, called an intraventricular haemorrhage and this can also cause anoxic brain damage.

These are four examples of how anoxic brain damage can occur at birth. If severe, the brain damage results in severe learning difficulties, cerebral palsy, epilepsy, or all three problems. However, it must be emphasized that most children with severe epilepsy and cerebral palsy will have had a normal birth and will not have suffered an anoxic brain injury. Other causes will be found to explain their epilepsy such as a brain malformation, a genetic disorder or an intrauterine infection.

A stroke is usually due to an obstruction to an artery that is supplying blood to a particular part of the brain. The nerve cells in the area of the brain supplied by the artery die as a result of lack of oxygen, or become damaged in such a way that they may form a focus for paroxysmal discharges later, and hence, may become a focus for epileptic seizures. Most strokes occur in late adult life, and cerebrovascular disease accounts for much of the epilepsy beginning in old age. Occasionally, however, a stroke may occur in a young adult or even in a child.

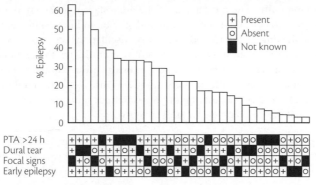

Figure 3.1 Incidence of late epilepsy after compound depressed fracture of the skull in which three or four factors were known. (Redrawn from W.B. Jennett [1975]. *Epilepsy after non-missile head injuries*. Heinemann, London, with kind permission.)

Very rarely, a prolonged febrile seizure (also called convulsion) which lasts 30 minutes or longer may also result in some anoxic damage. This damage is usually in one part of the brain, called the temporal lobe, which seems to be more vulnerable to anoxic damage particularly at the age when febrile seizures usually occur (between 12 months and 3 years of age. See Chapter 9).

Head injury

Damage to cerebral nerve cells may occur through physical trauma. In war time, (including terrorist attacks), head injuries due to penetrating injuries from shrapnel or bullets were a common and significant cause of epilepsy. About 45 per cent of survivors from such injuries develop epilepsy. In civilian life, most head injuries are closed—that is to say there is no penetration of the skull. However, the brain can be severely damaged in closed injuries and may result in epilepsy.

Studies undertaken many years ago have identified factors that are most likely to cause later epilepsy (Figure 3.1). These factors include the following:

♦ the duration of the post-traumatic amnesia (PTA), which is the name given to the period after a head injury when patients, although conscious, cannot remember or recall ongoing events from memory. A typical story is for a man to have no recollection of relatives visiting him in hospital in the days or weeks following the head injury, even though he talked and joked with them. The duration of post-traumatic amnesia may vary from a few minutes, when the term 'concussion' is often loosely applied, to many weeks or even months. The mechanism of the amnesia is not known, but a useful analogy is to consider a jelly in a mould (the brain in the skull). A vigorous tap or shaking of the mould may cause oscillations so violent within the jelly that cracks appear within its structure, even though the mould remains intact. Such vigorous forces can be demonstrated within the brains of animals subject to experimental head injuries. This is known as diffuse axonal injury. The longer the duration of post-traumatic amnesia, the greater is the chance of the development of later epilepsy.

◆ the presence of focal neurological signs after the injury, such as weakness of one side of the body or changes in the reflexes. This is simply because these focal signs reflect a greater degree of disruption of the brain.

◆ the presence of local damage to the cortical surface of the brain, as judged by the presence of a tear in the dura, i.e., the membrane covering the brain. The impact on the head from a sharp corner may cause a depressed fracture, with fragments of bone tearing the dura and becoming embedded in the underlying cerebral cortex (brain).

If all three factors were present in one case (a prolonged amnesia of more than 24 hours after the head injury, focal neurological signs, and a dural tear), then there was a 40 per cent chance of developing late, post-traumatic epilepsy. If none of these factors was present the risk was only about 2 per cent. This should be compared with the risk in the general population who have not had a severe head injury, when the risk is just less than 1 per cent.

Two other factors have been found to be associated with a higher risk of developing late epilepsy; these are early seizures and the level of unconsciousness or coma.

◆ it was also found that some head-injured patients had a seizure in the first week after the injury; these were called early seizures. The occurrence of an early seizure was a strong predictor of late post-traumatic epilepsy. This has been confirmed in more recent research undertaken in the last ten years. A seizure in the first week, accompanied by a long post-traumatic amnesia and focal neurological signs was followed by later seizures in 60 per cent of cases, even if the dura was not torn.

◆ a final factor that also been shown to predict the development of late, post-traumatic epilepsy is the severity of the level of consciousness or coma immediately after the head injury. This can be measured or scored using the Glasgow Coma Scale (GCS) which is a coma scale that is used throughout the world to assess the level of consciousness. Its name comes from Glasgow, the place where it was designed and first used by Professor Bryan Jennett. The normal score is 15; a GCS score of 8 or below has sometimes been found to be associated with a higher risk of late epilepsy.

Tumours

Brain tumours are rare, and have an incidence of around 10 per 100,000 per year. It is, however, true that tumours can cause epilepsy. This is much more likely to happen in adults than in children. Only about 1 per cent of all epilepsy in children is caused by a brain tumour. This is because brain tumours in children involve the brainstem and cerebellum, parts of the brain that do not give rise to seizures, and not the cerebral hemispheres.

Brain tumours are either primary or secondary. A secondary tumour is one that has been carried in the blood to the brain from another site. Cancers of the lung (bronchus) or breast are by far the most common of these. Usually the site of the original cancer is known, and the appearance of seizures in such a patient is an ominous sign indicating that a secondary tumour has arisen within the brain. Sometimes, however, the original cancer has not been discovered at the time of the first seizure, and a careful clinical examination will reveal a small tell-tale lump in the breast, or the lung cancer will be seen on an X-ray or computerized tomography (CT) scan of the chest.

Primary tumours of the brain do not usually arise in nerve cells. They either arise in the supporting cells between nerve cells, which play an active role in their nutrition (glial cells) or in the meninges, the covering membranes of the brain. These tumours are called gliomas and meningiomas. There are other types of primary cerebral tumours, such as those arising from the cells lining the cavities of the brain, or from blood vessels, but these are very rare. Primary brain tumours are not like cancer of the breast, or bowel, or bronchus. They show no tendency to develop blood-borne secondary deposits in other organs. This is fortunate, but there are other characteristics which prevent effective treatment.

- Gliomas infiltrate normal brains extensively, which can make complete surgical removal of the tumour very difficult. As a result, recurrence after surgical excision is common. These sorts of tumour are often treated with chemotherapy and radiotherapy as well as surgery.

- Meningiomas are encapsulated tumours, and can sometimes be removed completely, with a good chance of complete eradication. Unfortunately, meningiomas often have an extensive blood supply, so in some cases, complete removal may be technically very difficult or the operation may be complicated by a brain haemorrhage.

Infectious diseases

World-wide, particularly in the developing world, infectious diseases are a major cause of epilepsy as well as other neurological disabilities. Infections can arise from the following organisms:

- bacteria

- viruses

- protozoa

- parasites

- *Mycoplasma pneumoniae.*

Bacterial meningitis can damage the brain at any age from the newborn period to old age. Vigorous and early treatment with antibiotics and corticosteroid drugs (prednisolone or hydrocortisone) nearly always prevents damage to the cortex, which lies immediately under the meningeal covering of the brain. However, if the treatment is delayed, or the organism is resistant to the antibiotic chosen, the damaged cortical cells may act as seizure focus in subsequent years. Meningitis due to tuberculosis is particularly likely to result in later epilepsy. Meningitis caused by a virus tends to be a much milder illness and does not usually result in epilepsy.

A rarer brain infection caused by bacteria is a cerebral abscess. Bacteria usually arrive in the brain via the blood supply. This might occur in someone who is severely unwell with septicaemia, as well as in someone with a sinus or ear infection. Brain abscesses are also more common in people with congenital heart disease, sinus disease (sinusitis) and in those with unhealthy teeth. Patients with acute brain abscesses will commonly have seizures, and even if successfully treated by drainage and by antibiotics, over 40 per cent of individuals will go on to develop epilepsy.

Viral encephalitis occurs when a viral infection causes inflammation and damage to the brain, and this will commonly cause seizures. There are a large number of viruses that can cause encephalitis and some of these can be fatal, including rabies, measles, Western Nile virus, Japanese encephalitis and the herpes viruses. In the UK, two of the more common viruses causing encephalitis and seizures are the herpes and cytomegaloviruses. Cytomegalovirus usually affects the foetal (unborn baby's) brain through an intrauterine infection (the virus crossing the placenta and infecting the foetus). The herpes virus can affect people of any age, particularly if they have a depressed immune system which is not able to fight the virus. The HIV-AIDS virus can also cause seizures, either directly by itself or, indirectly by depressing the immune system, allowing invasion of the brain by other organisms including cytomegalovirus, tuberculosis and another organism called Toxoplasma, an organism known as a protozoon. Malaria, another protozoan infection, caused by *Plasmodium falciparum* and transmitted through mosquito bites can also cause severe encephalitis with frequent seizures.

Parasites can also cause epilepsy, more commonly in the developing world. The pork tapeworm *Taenia solium* may cause epilepsy if the cystic stage of the tapeworm, usually found in pigs, occurs in the brain of man. In developing countries, calcified cysts are found in the brains of many of the rural population and this disorder, cysticercosis, and tuberculosis account for a lot of the greater incidence of epilepsy in such populations. The dog tapeworm *Toxocara* has also been incriminated in the development of epilepsy, though with less certain evidence.

Acquired metabolic disorders

The pathways of chemical metabolism in the newborn are very unstable and large changes in the concentrations of various substances in the blood can occur. A blood glucose concentration sufficiently low (hypoglycaemia) to cause seizures, for example, cannot usually be induced in older children or adults by starvation, or indeed by any means other than the injection of insulin. However, severe hypoglycaemia resulting in seizures may be seen in:

◆ the newborn baby, particularly in premature infants

◆ babies born to diabetic mothers

◆ infants with rare metabolic defects, particularly when they are unwell with gastroenteritis, or if they are not able to eat and drink normally.

Other metabolic or biochemical disturbances may also cause seizures. These include low (or sometimes very high) levels of

◆ calcium (hypocalcaemia): one cause of a low blood calcium is feeding with cow's milk, which is very rich in phosphates. This results in increased loss of calcium through the kidneys and therefore low calcium levels in the blood. This is now an uncommon cause of seizures in UK, but still occurs in the developing countries

◆ sodium (low level, called hyponatraemia; high level, called hypernatraemia): these may result from severe and persistent vomiting or from endocrine (hormonal) disturbances in the body. This biochemical disturbance is again more likely to occur in infants and young children or following a severe head injury

◆ magnesium: low levels occur rarely and usually in people with serious disorders that affect the bowel or kidneys.

In adulthood, other acquired metabolic or biochemical disorders may cause seizures. These include hepatic (liver) and renal (kidney) failure. Chronic renal failure used to be one of the more common causes, but dialysis and successful transplantation of kidneys has reduced the frequency of seizures due to this cause.

> By definition, these seizures above are not epileptic seizures, but seizures caused by the metabolic or biochemical disturbance, which if treated, will prevent further seizures.

Alcohol

Alcohol may precipitate seizures in those who already have had previous seizures. This is discussed in Chapter 8. There is also an association between chronic alcohol abuse and the occurrence of fits even when the person is sober and not under the influence of alcohol. The most common type of seizure associated with alcohol is what is called an alcohol withdrawal seizure, which occurs when an alcoholic suddenly stops drinking for a few days. Seizures can also occur due to intoxication, after a period of binge drinking. In both situations, the seizures are directly due to the alcohol or its withdrawal. The person therefore does not have epilepsy and treatment with anti-epileptic drugs is not required, but the person will require treatment for the alcohol addiction.

People addicted to alcohol can also develop epilepsy for a number of reasons including:

◆ the effects of the chronic or long-term abuse of the alcohol on the brain

◆ people with an alcoholic addiction are more likely to have falls and sustain severe head injuries which can then cause epilepsy

◆ they may also start to abuse other recreational drugs, including ecstasy, cocaine and/or cannabis, which can also damage the brain.

In these circumstances, anti-epileptic drug treatment may be required in addition to treatment for the alcohol or other drug addiction, or both.

Table 3.2 Causes of epilepsy in two community studies (percent)

	USA	UK
Perinatal/congenital	8.0	–
Trauma	5.5	3.0
Vascular	10.9	15.0
Tumours	4.1	6.0
Infection	2.5	2.0
Degenerative	3.5	6.0
Alcohol	(excluded)	7.0
Uncertain (cryptogenic plus idiopathic)	65.5	61.0

USA Data from Olmstead County study (1993).
UK Data from National General Practitioner Study of Epilepsy (1990).
The most common degenerative disorder is Alzheimer's disease.

Degenerative disorders

Degenerative diseases that affect the cerebral cortex, such as Alzheimer's disease, Huntington's disease, some rare metabolic disorders (called mitochondrial disorders) and cerebral arteriosclerosis (hardening of the arteries of the brain) are associated with seizures. Seizures usually develop late in the course of these diseases.

How common are the individual causes of epilepsy?

Table 3.2 shows results from two studies, one from the UK and one from the USA. The researchers undertaking these studies tried to identify the causes of epilepsy in a particular group of patients. The table summarizes the causes that were found, but does not include a summary of those people who were likely to have a genetic cause for their epilepsy. Although the studies identified participants in different ways, the proportion for which a cause could be found was similar, between 34.5 and 39.0 per cent. Therefore, a cause was not found for around two-thirds of people with epilepsy. It is likely that a significant proportion of these people had a genetic cause for their epilepsy. Also, since these studies were undertaken there have been major advances in MRI imaging, and it is very likely, if not certain, that if these studies were repeated, a higher proportion of patients would be found to have structural abnormalities within their brain to explain the cause of their epilepsy.

Precipitants of seizures

Some things are known to precipitate or trigger seizures for people with epilepsy; the main precipitants or triggers are discussed below.

Sleep and lack of sleep

The relationship between sleep and seizures is complex and poorly understood. Sleep is a complex physiological process during which the brain goes through a number of stages or cycles. Some individuals will have all or virtually all their seizures whilst asleep. This is more common for people with focal or partial onset seizures.

Some people are more prone to seizures during the transition between sleep and wakefulness, and may have seizures when falling asleep or when waking. Seizures on or just after waking are more common, and this pattern is more commonly seen in people with an idiopathic generalized epilepsy (e.g. juvenile myoclonic epilepsy, or generalized epilepsy with tonic–clonic seizures on waking).

Sleep deprivation can trigger seizures. This occurs more often in people with one of the idiopathic generalized epilepsies and the seizure typically occurs the following morning. For young people, sleep deprivation often occurs whilst socializing, and at a time when alcohol might also be consumed. The combination of sleep deprivation and alcohol can be a very powerful trigger for seizures to occur. It is not uncommon for a teenager with epilepsy to have their first seizure following a night out socializing with friends.

Alcohol

Excess alcohol can trigger seizures in people with epilepsy, usually the following day. As discussed above, excess alcohol is often associated with sleep deprivation which can also trigger seizures. In addition, frequent and excessive alcohol intake can reduce the effectiveness of an individual's anti-epileptic medication, making it more likely for seizures to occur. When asked about alcohol consumption during clinic appointments, we discuss moderation in alcohol intake, rather than total abstinence. It is always difficult to define 'moderation' but this usually means no more than 2 units of alcohol on no more than two nights per week.

Menstruation and pregnancy

Women with epilepsy, especially those with focal onset seizures, may notice that their seizures cluster around the time of their menstrual periods; this is sometimes referred to as catamenial epilepsy. The precise reason for this occurrence is not known but may be due to the effect of sex hormones.

Seizures may also increase during pregnancy; up to one-third of women will report that their seizures have become more frequent during pregnancy and this may require a temporary change in the woman's anti-epileptic medication during her pregnancy. This may be particularly necessary for the anti-epileptic drug, lamotrigine.

Stress and worry

Some people notice that seizures are more likely at times of stress and worry. This is more common because stress and worry interfere with sleep, which as discussed, is a powerful trigger for provoking seizures. In addition, any alcohol and medication taken to try and reduce the stress and anxiety may also lower the threshold and increase the likelihood of experiencing a seizure. However, it is possible that in some people with epilepsy, stress and worry might also directly increase the risk of seizures.

Other illnesses

Any one with epilepsy may have a seizure in relation to a severe illness such as meningitis, encephalitis or severe gastroenteritis or pneumonia. In children with epilepsy, fever may increase the risk of seizures, but it is important to emphasize the difference between these and febrile seizures (convulsions) (Chapter 9).

Drugs

Some drugs increase the risk of seizures for people with epilepsy. This possible risk should be discussed before any new treatment is started, and this includes medicines bought over the counter in a pharmacy as well as for prescription drugs. Drugs that may make seizures worse include:

- anti-depressant drugs of the tricyclic group, including amitryptiline (for example, Tryptizol, Saroten, Dornical) and nortrypryline (for example, Allegron, Aventyl) and the selective serotonin uptake inhibitors (known as the SSRIs), including fluoxetine (Prozac) and paroxetine (Seroxat) have been associated with an increased risk of seizures, but this risk is probably small. However, it is important that depression in people with epilepsy is correctly recognized and appropriately treated.

- phenothiazines

- isoniazid

- clozapine

- high doses of penicillin and an antibiotic called ciprofloxacin

- some of the drugs to prevent malaria, called chloroquine and mefloquine.

> A number of other drugs may precipitate or trigger seizures in those with epilepsy and who are taking anti-epileptic medication by interfering with the metabolism of these drugs. Therefore, it is always important for someone with epilepsy, or their parents/carers, to ask the general practitioner or hospital specialist who prescribes another, non-epileptic drug or medicine, whether this new drug might interfere with their anti-epileptic medication or make their epilepsy worse, or both.

It should also be remembered that withdrawal of some drugs may precipitate seizures, particularly barbiturates or the benzodiazepines if they are withdrawn too quickly (over less than three months).

Finally, it is important to clarify one or two myths or misunderstandings about some other medicines or drugs that have been reported to make seizures worse in someone with epilepsy. The following drugs are *not* known to make seizures worse:

- stimulants such as methyphenidate (Ritalin or Equasym or Concerta) or atomoxetine (Strattera) used in children with attention deficit hyperactivity disorder (ADHD)

- all routine immunizations in childhood including the triple immunization (pertussis [whooping cough], diphtheria and tetanus), MMR (mumps, measles and rubella) meningococcal and haemophilus influenza vaccines and the BCG vaccine to protect against tuberculosis.

Toxins

A large number of toxins or poisons can also affect the brain and cause seizures. These include pesticides or some insecticides, and a range of chemicals.

However, once the individual is no longer exposed to the toxin and the source of the toxin is removed, the seizures should cease, unless the toxin has been poisonous enough to permanently damage the brain. This is very unlikely.

Other precipitants - reflex epilepsy

More specific than any of the precipitants so far discussed are the stimuli or triggers which result in what is called reflex epilepsy. There are many stimuli that can cause a reflex epilepsy, but by far the most common is that caused by lights that flash at a certain rate or frequency (usually between 14 and 30 flashes per second). Flashing lights of all colours may trigger a seizure but particularly those that are bright orange or red. This is called photosensitivity. Some young people have seizures induced by flashing lights, for example, in a night club or when travelling in a car when directly looking at a row of trees or railings in bright sunlight. Photosensitive epilepsy can be diagnosed on an EEG. In most people, an obvious pattern can be recorded from the back of the head (the occipital region) when a light is flashed in the eyes. With repeated flashes, these waves closely follow the flash frequency. At a critical frequency in a young person with photosensitive epilepsy, a totally different response occurs, as shown up on the EEG as multiple spikes and waves, known as polyspike and slow wave activity. This is called the photoparoxysmal response. Sometimes the person may also have a seizure in association with this photoparoxysmal response and this seizure may be either a myoclonic, or less commonly, a tonic–clonic seizure. Seizures may result, in photosensitive children and adults, from flickering light reflected from water, or by the interruption of steady light filtered through trees observed from a moving car. The most common stimulus to precipitate a seizure is the television or video or DVD games played on a personal computer (PC). This problem is primarily associated with the traditional TV rather than with flat screen LCD or plasma screen technology. Experiments have shown that it is the normal sweep or speed of the spots that make up the picture from side to side and down the face of the tube that causes the seizure, and not any malfunction of vertical picture or horizontal line hold. Susceptible children are most at risk when:

- the screen occupies a considerable proportion of the visual field, as will occur if the size of the screen is large, and the child sits close to it, or approaches it to change the programme.

- the child is tired or sleep-deprived. This is one of the reasons why photosensitivity is more likely to present for the first time in older children and teenagers who stay up late watching TV or playing computer games in their darkened bedrooms.

Therefore, the chances of a photically induced seizure are less likely to occur if:

- the person sits further away from the screen; it is recommended that they should sit at least three feet (one metre) away from the screen, whether it is a TV or computer screen

- the contrast is reduced between the screen and surroundings by placing the TV set or computer (PC) near a desk lamp or keeping an overhead light on in the room

- not playing the video or computer game when tired.

It has also been shown that the photoparoxysmal response cannot be elicited if only one eye is exposed to the flashing light. It makes sense, therefore, for susceptible children to cover one eye with a hand, if and when they approach the TV set. Changing channels using a remote control reduces the need to approach the TV. Both colour and monochrome television sets induce seizures, which are usually generalized, though they may sometimes be of very short duration—just a few myoclonic seizures affecting the patient's head, arm or trunk. Rarely, one or two myoclonic seizures may then progress to a tonic–clonic seizure. Although video or computer games may also precipitate or trigger seizures in people who are photosensitive, the text (words, figures and graphs) such as those found in Microsoft Word programmes, do not usually trigger seizures.

Another type of visual reflex epilepsy occurs on looking at patterns such as squares of floor tiling. This may be regarded as typical of the highly specific reflex epilepsies occurring in a very few patients. Other, very rare examples of reflex epilepsy include:

- reading (usually large print books or magazines)

- listening to certain types of music (this may be any type, including rock and pop, heavy metal, jazz, and classical and may involve only certain phrases or sections of the song or piece of music)

- performing mental arithmetic

- eating

- going into either hot or cold water (this very rare type usually only occurs in infants and children)

The perception of such external stimuli results in a very specific pattern of nerve cell activity that can trigger a seizure; how precisely this happens remains a mystery.

4

The first seizure and the diagnosis of epilepsy

⮕ Key points

♦ It is normal to experience a sense of shock, fear and panic upon seeing a tonic–clonic seizure for the first time.

♦ A person having a tonic–clonic seizure should be laid on their side in the recovery position only once the convulsion has stopped. Something soft should be put under their head. No attempt should be made to put anything in a person's mouth and between their teeth during a tonic–clonic seizure.

♦ If an ambulance is called, someone should try to accompany the person to hospital to provide moral support when recovery of consciousness occurs and also to give an accurate account of events to the hospital staff.

♦ It is very important to make sure that the history of events is as complete and as accurate as possible before a diagnosis of epilepsy is made. This includes asking about what the person was doing before the episode started, how it began, how it progressed, and how exactly it ended.

♦ If there is any doubt about the diagnosis of epilepsy, the person must be referred to a hospital specialist.

♦ There are many conditions other than epilepsy that can cause a person to fall down, jerk, twitch or lose consciousness.

Scenario one

Anyone, including doctors and nurses, who have been present for the first time at a tonic–clonic seizure of a child or adult will easily remember the feeling of shock, fear, and panic at coping with a totally unforeseen situation. A common story is for parents to be woken by the noisy breathing or grunting of a child in the next bedroom. They go to him, thinking usually that he is probably having a bad dream but may find him:

- staring

- unresponsive

- convulsing

- his mouth 'frothing'

- perhaps blue

- blood on the pillow because the tongue or inside of the cheek has been bitten

Few if any parents can cope calmly with such a scene. The immediate response is usually to panic and do nothing, or do something that is inappropriate and potentially dangerous.

> They should never try to put something between his teeth—this is a very dangerous thing to do that may damage the person's teeth and also result in a bitten finger for the person who is trying to put something in their mouth.

Alternatively, they may run next door for help, particularly if they live next door to a nurse or doctor. Finally, they may ring the out-of-hours doctor (general practitioner) or NHS Direct or telephone 999 for an ambulance. Sometimes parents may do some or all of these things simultaneously!

Almost invariably, however, by the time the out-of-hours GP or ambulance has arrived, the seizure is over, and the child may be asleep or awake but confused, possibly having vomited. The parents are likely to be afraid and anxious, as they might have thought that he was going to die, or that another convulsion was about to begin. It is unlikely that they will be able to sleep; even if their son then falls into a deep sleep and doesn't wake up until the following afternoon.

Scenario two

Although the first seizure can occur anywhere and at any time, another common scenario is for the first seizure to occur in a young woman in the company of her friends or at work. In this case, the lack of immediate or easy access to the general practitioner, whose name and telephone number is unlikely to be known by anyone around her, results in an ambulance being called, and the young woman is then rushed off to hospital. She will recover consciousness either in the ambulance or in the accident and emergency department of the hospital. When she comes round she will always be confused and this will be made worse by the feeling of, 'What is going on; why am I on a stretcher (or on a hospital trolley or bed) with strangers staring at me or doing things to me?'

In this situation, although ambulance services are rather uncomfortable about allowing it, a friend should be allowed to accompany her to hospital not only to provide moral support when recovery of consciousness occurs, but also to give an accurate account of events to the hospital staff. In this case, the diagnosis of a tonic–clonic seizure is clear, but in others, the situation may not be that clear, particularly if the seizure was a focal (complex partial) seizure.

It is obviously very important to distinguish between an epileptic seizure and some other event which may initially seem to be one. Patients, or more commonly their parent, friend or just a bystander who saw the episode, may speak in terms of the person having a blackout, funny turn, or blank spell, or a fit, and the medical staff have to do their best to try and work out exactly what happened in this blackout or fit, and whether it might have been an epileptic seizure.

What will the family doctor (GP) or accident and emergency doctor do?

Apart from listening carefully to the story given by the person and any eyewitness who had seen the seizure or other event(s), the doctor will also examine the patient.

The examination

They will examine her patient not only to make sure that everything is generally well, for example, that his breathing is unobstructed, but will also try and find out:

- whether the person has a high temperature (particularly if the person is a young child)

- whether the tongue has been bitten

- whether they have been incontinent

- whether there are any focal (localized) neurological signs, which may give her a clue to the cause of the seizure

- whether there may be any birth marks such as white or coffee-coloured marks which might indicate a condition that might be linked with epilepsy (such as tuberous sclerosis or neurofibromatosis).

Though she is not likely to find anything abnormal at this stage, there may be some minor signs such as an asymmetry of the reflexes. She will then talk to the relatives or any other witnesses, and try and satisfy herself that what has just occurred was indeed an epileptic seizure, and not some other event of the type discussed later in this chapter.

Rarely, the first seizure is an early manifestation of an acute and important illness such as meningitis or encephalitis, particularly in children, or a head injury, and it is always important to consider this possibility in infants and toddlers. If she suspects that this might be the case, she will, of course, arrange immediate admission to hospital for specialist advice and investigation.

Medication

If the person is still convulsing—or another convulsion starts in the surgery or in the accident and emergency department—then it may be necessary to give some emergency (also called rescue) medication to stop the seizure. In the surgery, this will usually be midazolam, which is gently squirted into the cheek (called the buccal cavity) or, less commonly, diazepam which is gently squirted up the rectum (back passage). If the person is in the accident and emergency department then it is possible that instead of midazolam, they may be given an intravenous injection of diazepam or lorazepam. Whatever is given is likely to reduce the chance that another tonic–clonic seizure will occur within the next 12 to 24 hours, although unfortunately, this can never be guaranteed.

In most situations, if the person has had to be given some emergency medication, and particularly if this was a child, then they will need to be admitted to hospital, even for a brief period of observation. This will ensure that the person recovers fully and also does not go on to have another tonic–clonic convulsion. It also gives people time to collect their thoughts and decide on what should happen next—which could include decisions about further tests, whether to refer to a specialist and whether the person needs to be started on an anti-epileptic treatment.

Is referral to a specialist necessary?

A specialist is usually defined as a hospital doctor.

- For children, the hospital specialist can be a paediatrician or a paediatric neurologist who has specific training and an interest in treating children with epilepsy.

- For adults (anyone over 16 or 17 years of age), the specialist will be an adult physician or neurologist. When the specialist *only* sees patients with epilepsy, they are often called an epileptologist.

Some referrals to a hospital specialist are because the general practitioner (GP) is unclear as to whether the person has had an epileptic seizure. However, where episodes occur in a child or teenager, then most GPs will refer them to a paediatrician or paediatric neurologist, even when the GP thinks that the episodes have been epileptic seizures. This is because children may experience many different types of episodes or funny turns that may not be epileptic seizures and it is therefore important to make the correct diagnosis. It is particularly important to make a correct diagnosis before any treatment is prescribed. In most situations, referral to a hospital specialist is usually for the following reasons:

- People or parents do not like being told that they—or their child—have had an epileptic seizure. One survey showed that this difficult task is left to the hospital doctor in about half the cases.

- People with epilepsy themselves very often feel that some sort of special test is necessary to prove the diagnosis. This point is discussed in relation to the EEG in Chapter 5. It is often very difficult to accept the diagnosis, with all its social implications, when it is made on the basis of a 30-second description given to a doctor by a relative or bystander. Somehow it does not seem scientific enough; yet paediatricians and neurologists place enormous weight on the recounted stories. This is entirely justified because it is important to understand that the diagnosis of an epileptic seizure and epilepsy is nearly always made on the basis of a very detailed story (called the history) and the hospital specialist will always have more time than the GP to take a detailed history.

◆ People with epilepsy are very concerned to discover the cause of their epilepsy. As Table 3.2 shows, a cause is often not found, but most people think in terms of a single cause, which they believe, if found and treated (or removed), will result in the problem (the epilepsy) being sorted out once and for all. Sometimes an important treatable cause *is* found, and usually special tests are necessary to show this, such as a brain scan. The difficulty usually lies in deciding which patients should be so investigated.

◆ Medical textbooks and even the Internet often focus on and emphasize the unusual and interesting causes of epilepsy, often at the expense of the more usual patients. General practitioners often decide to play it safe and refer the person in to the nearest referral centre.

◆ The necessary decisions are quite complex. There are three possible preliminary diagnoses:

   ◆ a definite epileptic seizure

   ◆ not an epileptic seizure

   ◆ possibly an epileptic seizure.

Once the history is taken, the next decision is—what if any investigations need to be arranged; after that the next decision is—whether medication is or is not indicated and whether simply to adopt a wait-and-see policy; the final decision that may then need to be taken is whether the person needs to be referred to another specialist, one who only treats individuals with epilepsy (the epileptologist). In view of these potential decisions—and trying to make the right decision—it is often wise for the GP or family doctor to refer the person to a hospital specialist. Certainly, if the GP is uncertain about the nature or diagnosis of the person's funny turn or blackout, they should, if not *must*, refer them in to obtain a correct diagnosis.

What will the paediatrician, paediatric neurologist or neurologist do?

The analysis of funny turns or blackouts of one sort or another makes up a considerable proportion of the work of a neurologist and quite a bit of the work of a paediatrician or paediatric neurologist Their first concern is to obtain as accurate as possible an account of the events which led up to and occurred at the time of a seizure. People who have lost consciousness cannot themselves say what happened while they were unconscious.

However, people will be able to give important information about what they were doing at the time of the episode and how they felt before loss of consciousness, and how they felt when they first recovered, but the neurologist will want to know what was happening before, during and throughout the time that consciousness was disturbed. For this reason an eye-witness account is crucial. Information must be asked about:

- what time of day was it?

- what was the person doing before the attack?

- what were the events leading up to the seizure(s)?

- did the seizure or attack occur without warning, or were there initial symptoms suggestive of an aura, or of a simple faint (syncope) (see later in this chapter)?

- what precisely did the child or person look like or do during the seizure?

- how long did the seizure or attack last?

- how did the seizure stop?

- what did the person look like and do afterwards?

- when was the person back to being completely 'normal'?

If the patient or eye-witness is unable to recall accurately exactly what happened during the seizure, then it is useful and important to ask the eye-witness to show the doctor what sort of 'jerking' or 'shaking' or 'twitching' occurred, although sometimes people are too shy or embarrassed to do this. In these situations we will often try and mime what they are describing and then ask them to tell us if this is what they saw! If repeated attacks occur, and the diagnosis remains unclear or difficult, the potential eye-witness should be given a list of the things to look out for and also encouraged to use a video-camera or camcorder. Even mobile phones can be used to record a person's episodes and we have certainly been able to make a diagnosis of not only epileptic seizures but also simple faints or mannerisms (also called 'tics') from the video recorded on a mobile phone. Children's schools can also be encouraged to video the child's episodes if they occur at school, providing the families give their consent for this practice.

Video-recordings have proved very useful in the diagnosis of epilepsy, particularly in infants and young children.

The diagnosis

It should be possible to make a definite diagnosis of epilepsy or of some other condition on the basis of all this clinical information. The diagnosis of epilepsy must not be made lightly and if there is doubt then epilepsy should *not* be diagnosed and the doctor should wait for more definite or convincing evidence from further attacks or episodes before making a firm diagnosis. The risk of someone with epilepsy coming to harm from a delay in the diagnosis is small, whereas a diagnosis of epilepsy incorrectly made is nearly always damaging. This damage may be reflected in unfair prejudice and resulting social and educational or employment restrictions, in addition to the prescription of unnecessary and potentially hazardous medication.

Conditions misdiagnosed as epilepsy

A large number of conditions may be misdiagnosed as epilepsy particularly in children. These include:

Simple faints (syncope; vasovagal attacks)

The medical name for these is syncope. Many of us have experienced one or more syncopal attacks, very often at school. In syncope, consciousness is disturbed or lost, not because of an abnormal discharge of nerve cells in the brain, but because these nerve cells are affected by an inadequate supply of oxygen to the brain.

What causes syncope?

When a person stands up, their brain is about 15 inches (38 cm) higher than their heart; when they lie down, the two organs are at the same level. When they stand up, therefore, the arterial blood pressure has to increase so that blood flow to the brain remains unchanged. Normally, this is accomplished smoothly by a combination of increased heart rate and by constriction of the blood vessels in the abdomen and legs. This regulatory mechanism can stop working in a number of situations. The most common is the extreme slowing of the heart-rate produced in some sensitive people by the sight of blood or in response to pain or a sudden shock. This cardiac slowing is mediated through the vagal nerve, and the name vasovagal attack is often given to such an episode.

Table 4.1 The usual differences between syncope and seizures

	Syncope	Seizures (tonic–clonic)
Posture	Upright usually	Any posture
Pallor and sweating	Invariable	Uncommon
Onset	Gradual	Usually sudden
Injury	Rare	Not uncommon
Single jerks	Common, but brief	Common
Convulsions	Uncommon	Common
Incontinence	Unusual	Common
Tongue-biting	Rare	Common
Unconsciousness	Seconds	Minutes
Recovery	Rapid	Often slow
Post-ictal sleep	Rare	Common
Post-ictal confusion	Rare	Common
Precipitating factors	Crowded places; lack of food; sudden pain, fright or shock	Rare

The contraction of leg and thigh muscles during walking normally sends venous blood back to the heart. If venous blood return is insufficient because of immobility—for example, a person standing for some time in a hot, crowded train or bus, or a young girl in assembly at school—then syncope is likely to occur. Such syncope is occasionally socially infectious, and once a girl or woman has collapsed or fainted, others may follow in the next few minutes.

Normally blood returns to the heart from the legs smoothly through the chest and abdomen. During prolonged coughing, or straining while trying to pass water or faeces (as when constipated), the pressure within the chest is greatly increased, preventing venous return to the heart. What the heart is not getting back, it cannot put out, so this sequence of events again usually results in impaired blood flow to the brain—and syncope.

If the blood vessels in the torso (trunk of the body) and legs are pleasantly dilated in a hot bath or nice warm bed, suddenly getting up—for example, to answer the telephone—may also cause syncope. This may also happen in older people, when they get out of bed at night to pass urine. The situation is more complex in this case because we know that, at the onset of urination, there is a reflex dilatation of blood vessels in the legs. This so-called micturition syncope affects men more than women, not only because they more often have to pass urine at night (because of prostatic enlargement) but because they pass urine standing up.

Syncope may occur in association with certain diseases. For example, in diabetes the nerve fibre controlling the heart rate and the diameter of blood vessels may be diseased, and the normal adjustments to blood pressure to posture may fail to occur. There are other rare diseases of the brain in which a similar failure to control blood pressure occurs. One very rare disease, which bears some similarity to Parkinson's disease, is known as the Shy–Drager syndrome after the two American neurologists who first described it.

A much more common cause of syncope, however, is medication. Many people take tablets to control high blood pressure. One effect of some of these drugs is to cause syncope on standing up. Some anti-depressants, such as imipramine (Tofranil), have the same effect.

Diagnosis of syncope

How does the neurologist or paediatrician decide that his patient's blackouts are due to syncope rather than epilepsy? The answer is in the story—or medical history. The first clue would be the circumstances in which the funny turn or blackout occurred. If it happened at the scene of a road accident, or hearing bad news, or in a girl or woman during a heavy menstrual period, or at a time when someone has been standing up for some time, syncope is very likely. A common story is for a man to faint while attending his wife's delivery or even when he is having his blood taken. This is more likely to occur in very fit or athletic men who tend to have a very low heart rate.

Syncope can, but hardly ever occurs lying down, so if loss of consciousness happens then, a seizure is more likely. Very occasionally, vagal slowing of the heart can be so profound that syncope *does* happen lying down. For example, one of our patients was a woman who was so terrified of dental treatment that she lost consciousness due to syncope even if the dentist treated her with the chair tilted back almost to the horizontal position.

Another useful feature that is helpful in making a diagnosis of syncope is the occurrence of pre-syncopal symptoms. Blood flow to the brain is reduced in syncope, often for many seconds before consciousness is lost. During that time, the nervous system makes desperate attempts to constrict other blood vessels in order to elevate the central pressure. This can result in the following:

- the constriction of blood vessels in the skin results in an extreme pale or ashen grey colour, often described as the person looking deathly white.

- there may also be the associated discharge of the vegetative (non-voluntary) nervous system—the autonomic nervous system—which results in the person becoming nauseated and sweaty, what is often called a cold sweat.

- the pupils of their eyes may also become dilated.

Therefore, in summary, the person who is about to faint, feels cold, clammy and dizzy and looks pale and 'not quite with it', may be having syncopal symptoms rather than epilepsy or seizure symptoms.

Other points which may help to distinguish syncope from seizures include:

- limpness, rather than rigidity

- brief jerks during the period of unconsciousness

- no incontinence during the event

- a relatively rapid recovery.

Recovery of full consciousnesss and orientation is much more rapid after syncope than after a seizure, following which there is usually a period of confusion and often a severe, throbbing headache. Recovery after syncope often rapidly follows assumption of the horizontal position, whether the person falls, or is placed so that the head is on the same level as the heart. This is nature's safety mechanism whereby cerebral blood flow is restored. Occasionally, the safety mechanism cannot operate—as in the position of a hand-basin or lavatory preventing the person's limp or stiff body falling to the floor. Sometimes the sufferer is supported in a vertical position by well-meaning but ill-advised friends or bystanders. This is more likely to occur in children, where a parent or an older sibling tries to comfort the child by holding them upright in their arms. In these cases, cerebral blood flow may fall to such extremely low levels that incontinence, twitching, or a full-blown seizure may occur. This should be regarded as an anoxic seizure rather than a seizure caused by epilepsy.

As an example of the difficulties that this unusual sequence of events can cause, one of us was asked to see a young nurse. Three days after a straightforward operation to remove her appendix, she got up for the first time to go to the bathroom. She felt faint as she walked there, and therefore left the door slightly open. She felt fainter still as she was sitting on the seat, straining to open her bowels. Before losing consciousness, she called another nurse for help. This girl seeing her colleague about to fall off the seat, held her up to prevent injury. The resulting cerebral anoxia caused an anoxic seizure. An incorrect diagnosis of epilepsy had been made, and her continued employment as a nurse was under threat. Fortunately, because we were able to obtain a full account of the sequence of the events we were able to 'unmake' the diagnosis of epilepsy.

Syncope in adolescents

Unfortunately this is a relatively common event and one of us has been involved in two legal cases where teenage girls were incorrectly diagnosed as having epilepsy because of episodes that were almost identical to those described above; on both occasions the syncope had been precipitated by very painful and heavy menstrual periods during which both girls had collapsed and then 'jerked' for a few seconds.

Syncope in adolescents—usually girls—can be very troublesome, and occasionally an injury can occur. Physique and lifestyle seem irrelevant, so the usual advice to take plenty of fresh air and exercise is probably useless. Much more important is to tell the young person to sit down with their head between their knees, or if possible, to lie down *at once* if they feel the onset of typical pre-syncopal symptoms. Fortunately recurrent episodes are rarely troublesome for more than a year. If syncopal attacks continue to occur, even after very minor triggers, a small amount of extra salt can be taken regularly in the diet. Rarely for troublesome syncope, some medication such as a very mild steroid can be prescribed to make this less likely to happen.

Reflex anoxic seizures

These are a type of syncope, but deserve a particular mention as the attacks are frequently misdiagnosed as epileptic seizures. Reflex anoxic seizures (also called pallid syncopal attacks) usually affect young children between 12 months and 4 years of age, but can affect older children and even adults. The attacks are *always* provoked by either a sudden fright, or unexpected pain. The pain often follows a bang on the back of the head or trapping a finger or toe in a drawer or door; it can also follow having an injection, for instance, when the child has an immunization or blood test. This unpleasant experience then stimulates a nerve (the vagus nerve) which causes the heart to slow down or even stop for a few seconds. The child may cry for a few seconds but then stops, becomes pale, then limp, and may even have a brief clonic convulsion lasting a few seconds but never more than a minute. Almost immediately the child will recover, may cry, and then appear sleepy. Within a few minutes the child is usually back to normal. These attacks do not damage the brain or heart, do not need treatment, and usually stop by the age of 5–10 years. When they persist into adulthood, the episodes can look very like syncopal or vasovagal attacks.

Breath-holding attacks

These attacks occur only in young children, aged usually between 1 and 3 years. The typical story is of a child who is frustrated, told off, or spanked or smacked. The child becomes angry or upset, cries vigorously for many seconds and eventually is not able to catch their breath. After a few seconds the child becomes blue (cyanosed) because of a lack of oxygen in the blood, loses consciousness, and becomes limp. Because of the reduced oxygen supply to the brain (as the child is not breathing) the child may become stiff and then have some isolated myoclonic or repeated clonic (jerking) movements and may even wet themselves. The child always starts breathing again and is back to normal within a few minutes. These breath-holding attacks usually stop by the age of 4–5 years. Sometimes these episodes are provoked or triggered by a painful event and the child can look as though they are having a reflex anoxic seizure.

Other causes of impaired oxygen supply to the brain

Disturbances of cardiac rhythm (cardiac arrhythmia)

Disturbance of consciousness in syncope is due to failure of blood supply to the brain, due in part to a fall in cardiac output. Cardiac output may also be less than normal if the rhythm of the heart is abnormal. Both very slow and very fast heart rates can reduce the cardiac output.

Distinguishing a disturbance of consciousness caused by an abnormality of cardiac rhythm from an epileptic seizure is not easy—but is extremely important—because the treatments and outcomes are very different.

Occasionally however, an observer may have found that someone is pulse-less or has a very irregular pulse during the attack, and sometimes the sufferer himself notices palpitations before the blackout and loss of consciousness. Cardiac rhythm is easily monitored by electrocardiography (an ECG). The changes in voltage associated with contraction of the different chambers of the heart are of sufficient amplitude that they can easily be recorded on a cassette recorder for periods of 24 hours, and, if necessary, over many days or even weeks and their occurrence in relation to symptoms then analyzed. A cardiac cause for disturbance of consciousness has been found in up to one quarter of cases first presenting to neurological clinics with blackouts. The most common cardiac arrhythmia that may cause blackouts is the prolonged QT interval syndrome, a condition which may be inherited and run in families; this condition may also be associated with deafness. The prolonged QT syndrome is diagnosed by doing an electrocardiogram (ECG) test. However, there are many other types of cardiac arrhythmias.

The important features that should result in a doctor thinking that a cardiac arrhythmia has caused a blackout are the following:

◆ where the episodes have occurred during or immediately after a vigorous period of exercise—swimming, running or cycling or the exercises that are frequently linked with triggering a cardiac arrhythmia

◆ when the episode has occurred after a sudden shock or surprise

◆ when the person's lips become cyanosed (blue)

◆ when the person falls stiffly rather than falling limply.

Clearly some of the above features may also be seen in reflex anoxic seizures, although reflex anoxic seizures are more commonly seen in infants and young children whereas a cardiac arrhythmia is more commonly seen in teenagers and adults. Whenever there is *any* doubt about the possibility of a cardiac arrhythmia causing a blackout or funny turn, or a drop seizure then an electrocardiogram (ECG) must be undertaken or the person should be referred to a specialist in heart disease (a cardiologist). There is no doubt that many people with a cardiac arrhythmia have been wrongly diagnosed as having epilepsy. Most cardiac arrhythmias can be treated with medication or a pacemaker. Importantly, failure to correctly diagnose a cardiac arrhythmia may result in severe brain injury and death.

Localized reduction in cerebral blood flow

The changes in blood flow that we have discussed so far affect all parts of the brain equally. In older people, atherosclerotic changes take place in the arteries in the neck and head (atherosclerosis is often known as hardening of the arteries). There may be a temporary blockage of an artery to one part of the brain by a fragment of chalky deposit or thrombus swept downstream from a larger artery by the flow of blood. Neurologists call these blockages transient ischaemic attacks. In some of these short episodes, muscle weakness or tingling in one or other limb may slightly resemble partial motor or sensory seizures (Chapter 2). However, although focal motor seizures may arise in the scarred brain in the territory of a permanently blocked artery after a stroke, transient ischaemic attacks are associated with transient paralysis rather than convulsions. Where the blockage in blood flow is more serious, the result may be a stroke or seizure, including tonic–clonic seizures that may occur at the time of the stroke. Seizures are far more likely when the stroke has occurred because of a bleeding from, rather than a blockage of, a blood vessel in the brain. This is called a haemorrhagic stroke.

In younger people, localized (focal) neurological phenomena occur in migraine. In the first stage of a classical migraine attack, arterial spasm occurs, reducing cerebral blood flow focally. It is unclear whether this is primary or secondary to some depression of nerve cell activity. The occipital lobe of the brain is the region most often affected. This results in a hallucination of distorted vision or flashing lights, rather than the formed visual hallucination which may be part of a partial seizure arising in a temporal lobe (Chapter 2). In migraine, this is called the aura, and the flashing lights are usually bright white or silver and are jagged or zigzag lines. Sometimes, they are likened to the appearance of the trenches of the First World War seen from the air (called fortification spectra) or the walls on the top of castles. Occasionally, the blood vessel spasm affects the motor or sensory areas of the brain, producing short-lived paralysis or disturbance of sensation, without convulsions, on the opposite side of the body; this is called hemiplegic migraine.

Narcolepsy

This is an uncommon condition, particularly in children, but may be misdiagnosed as epilepsy. The condition has four characteristic features:

- falling asleep frequently, in any situation and often suddenly

- cataplexy—falling down as if suddenly paralysed

- sleep paralysis—not being able to move yet fully conscious when falling asleep

- hypnagogic hallucinations (hallucinations while falling asleep)

However, most people with narcolepsy have only the first two or three of these features. All of us, at one time or another, will feel drowsy in a stuffy lecture theatre, or as a passenger on a long car journey—and may even fall asleep. People who suffer from narcolepsy, however, feel an uncontrollable desire to sleep at other times, and may indeed fall asleep in any situation and at any time, including in socially embarrassing circumstances. The periods of sleep may last minutes to over an hour and they don't always feel refreshed and fully awake afterwards. This unusual symptom may be associated with cataplexy—a sudden loss of postural tone causing collapse and becoming limp without any loss of consciousness. These episodes of cataplexy are nearly always provoked or triggered by strong emotions such as shock, anger or laughter. In a way, these phenomena are nearest to epilepsy, as they presumably result from some paroxysmal disorder of cerebral nerve cells. Again, it is very important to ask whether the episodes of 'collapse' (the cataplexy) are unprovoked or provoked—and obtaining the information that they *only* occur when triggered or provoked should lead to the correct diagnosis. Two other features may also occur in narcolepsy—sleep paralysis and hypnagogic (meaning 'as one falls asleep') hallucinations. In sleep paralysis, which can be very frightening, the person is awake but is unable to move. The episodes usually occur as the person is falling asleep or when they suddenly wake having been asleep for a short time. In hypnagogic hallucinations, the person experiences vivid and often frightening hallucination or bad dream-like feelings, again, as they are about to fall asleep. Narcolepsy can occur at any age—even in young children—but is more likely to occur and be diagnosed in late childhood and early adult life. Individuals with narcolepsy do not experience epileptic seizures any more often than the general population, the EEG whilst awake is usually normal, and drugs of a completely different type from those used in epilepsy may be effective in reducing or stopping both the periods of uncontrollable sleep and cataplexy.

Drop attacks

These nearly always affect only middle-aged women, and then often only for a year or two. The story is quite striking. The person complains that, while walking along, she suddenly finds that her legs have given way. She may land on her knees or pitch forward on her face. In either case, she is always adamant that she is fully aware of what is happening, and equally adamant that she did not trip over anything. The condition is variously assumed to be due to some weakness of the thigh muscles, or to a disturbance of blood flow in the brainstem, interfering with the postural reflexes that keep us upright. Whatever the mechanism, it is clear that these episodes are not a type of epileptic seizure.

Jumping legs or arms (nocturnal myoclonus, also called hypnic jerks)

About 80 per cent of adults (possibly more) will, at some time in their lives, experience sudden jerk of one or other leg, usually in the twilight stage of drifting off to sleep. The jerk is associated with, or may cause, a sudden arousal or awakening. Some people have a great number of jerks, so many that their wife, husband or partner, being bruised by the kicks, will refuse to share a bed with them. These jerks almost certainly represent some sort of paroxysmal discharge of nerve cells, probably in the brainstem (the part of the brain that connects the brain with the spinal cord) and not in the brain. They are therefore not an epileptic seizure, because epileptic seizures arise from the brain, and specifically the cerebral hemispheres. Other evidence that would support the belief that these hypnic jerks are not a type of epileptic seizure is because they occur in most adults and only in a specific situation, when drifting off to sleep. In addition, the jerks are never followed immediately by a tonic–clonic seizure. Importantly, these hypnic jerks or nocturnal myoclonus are not related to the jerks or myoclonic seizures that are associated with juvenile myoclonic epilepsy or juvenile-onset absence epilepsy (Chapter 2).

Vertigo

Doctors are careful to distinguish true vertigo—a perception of disequilibrium of the body in its relation to space—from non-specific feelings in the head such as 'dizziness' or 'muzziness' which are very often associated with anxiety, depression or the chronic fatigue syndrome. Vertigo is usually described by sufferers as:

◆ 'the room spinning around'

◆ 'as though I am always falling to one side'.

For obvious reasons, children often find it very difficult to use this description and will simply say that they feel dizzy. They might also look frightened or unwell and may run to a parent or look very pale and then vomit. True vertigo is only rarely a symptom of a focal (partial) seizure arising from one of the temporal lobes. In addition, the person whose episodes of vertigo are due to a focal seizure will almost always be experiencing other and much more easily recognizable epileptic seizures. Far more commonly, vertigo is due to a disorder of the balancing organ—the labyrinth—which lies within the inner ear. The labyrinth may malfunction in an episodic way in both children and adults. This is very likely to happen in someone who has an ear or bad upper respiratory tract infection. Sometimes, and particularly in young children, the distinction between paroxysmal vertigo and partial seizures may not be easy, as in both the child is frightened, and may either hold on to his parent or fall. The distinction rests on the absence of amnesia or confusion after the attack of benign paroxysmal vertigo and the fact that children will usually fall asleep after a focal seizure, even if it only lasts one or two minutes. When there is any doubt, tests of labyrinthine function will usually confirm true vertigo and exclude focal epilepsy.

Rigors

Occasionally the shivering associated with high fever, particularly frequent in infections of the urinary tract or kidney, may be confused with a tonic–clonic convulsion. Again, this is more likely to cause confusion in infants and children. We have lost count of the number of young children (and some adults) with rigors who have been wrongly diagnosed of having had a tonic–clonic convulsion.

Night terrors

These episodes are common in children between the ages of 4 and 10 years and frequently worry parents. Typically, a child who has been in bed, asleep for between 30 and 90 minutes will waken suddenly, screaming. They will be sitting up in bed, wide-eyed and unresponsive; they may thrash around and cannot be comforted. Within five, ten or occasionally fifteen minutes, sometimes a little longer, the child will lie down, turn over, and go back to sleep. There is no memory or recollection of the event the next morning and they awake, refreshed, as if nothing had happened the night before. These episodes only occur once a night and may occur nightly for some nights and then stop. Reassurance (of the parents) is all that is required. Sometimes, focal (partial) seizures arising from the frontal lobes may look a little like a night terror. However, in focal seizures the following usually occur:

◆ they are nearly always of shorter duration (only one to three minutes)

◆ they have bizarre posture of an arm or leg or the entire side of the body, called dystonia

◆ they usually occur more than once a night, even up to three, four or more times a night

◆ they occur repeatedly, night after night

Taking a video of the episodes may prove to be very helpful if the doctor finds it difficult to differentiate between night terrors and frontal lobe focal seizures.

Rage attacks/outbursts of temper

Bizarre, semi-purposeful behaviour and episodes of agitation or confusion may rarely be part of a complex partial seizure arising from one of the temporal lobes. Sometimes people can be confused after an epileptic seizure and if they are approached by someone trying to help them, they may think that they are being attacked and become aggressive. This is often called post-ictal (post-seizure) rage. However, violent behaviour or uncontrolled outbursts of rage themselves are almost *never* a type of epileptic seizure. If the story is properly taken, it becomes clear that the episodes are nearly always provoked, even by fairly minor events, such as someone changing a TV programme without asking or even looking at them the 'wrong way'. In addition, the rage is usually very obviously directed at someone or something, which is not the case when rage or agitation occurs as part of an epileptic seizure. The outbursts of rage may be quite violent and may last minutes or even up to half an hour or longer. After the longer ones, the person may be confused, exhausted, and then fall asleep. Sometimes when they wake up, they cannot recall what they had said or done—even if they had wrecked furniture or broken windows. It is these features of confusion, sleeping and amnesia for the event that often lead to a wrong diagnosis of epilepsy. This condition is often called the episodic dyscontrol syndrome, because the person periodically or episodically loses control. Finally, although rarely rage or agitation may be due to a partial (focal) seizure, these people nearly always already have a diagnosis of epilepsy and have more easily recognizable seizures, including focal (complex partial) seizures and even secondarily generalized tonic–clonic seizures.

Tics, habits, and ritualistic movements

Tics, also sometimes called *mannerisms*, are common in children, particularly boys and usually start around 6 or 7 years of age, sometimes younger. The tics usually involve the upper part of the face like screwing up the eyes, rapid blinking or a flick of the head. More complex habits such as grunting, sniffing and brushing the hair away from the eyes are common in children, and are rarely confused with seizures. If the tic is really complex and involves movements and sudden noises or words (called vocal tics), and has been present for more than a year or so, it is possible that the child may have something called Tourette syndrome. Children with Tourette syndrome may also have other mannerisms including ritualistic or obsessive traits and learning difficulties. It is unusual for children to have both epilepsy and Tourette syndrome.

Masturbation or self-gratification

It is quite common for children to indulge in strange patterns of movement which they find pleasurable, and which they stop immediately, either when they realize they are being watched or when they are told off. Sometimes infants and toddlers will rock backwards and forwards squeezing their thighs together and sometimes going red in the face—to the point where they appear to be masturbating. This is also called self-gratification. This is quite normal behaviour in young children, affecting girls and boys fairly equally, and is most often seen when they are tired or bored. Occasionally, they will be so engrossed or preoccupied in this activity that it may take a few seconds to get their attention. It is this feature that may convince some parents, and even doctors, that the child is having a complex partial or an absence seizure.

Colic

Colic or wind is a very common symptom in babies and young infants, and is usually easily recognized and diagnosed. However, occasionally infantile spasms (West syndrome), may be mistaken for colic or some other type of pain, which can lead to a delay in the diagnosis of this type of epilepsy. In colic, the child will be screaming fairly constantly and will be very restless. In children who are having infantile spasms, the child may be restless and then suddenly his arms or legs or both will jerk inwards or outwards (this is the spasm) for 2–4 seconds after which the child will appear distressed and cry. If the child has another spasm whilst crying, then the cry will suddenly stop; only to start again after the spasm has stopped. This cycle can then be repeated for a few minutes and occasionally for up to half an hour. There should really be no difficulty in distinguishing infantile spasms from colic.

Over-breathing

Breathing in and out too fast and too deep, like palpitations, is one bodily way in which anxiety, is manifested. This response seems to be particularly common in adolescent girls. If continued for more than a few minutes, excessive carbon dioxide is removed by the lungs from the blood, which becomes correspondingly alkaline. This may temporarily reduce the level of calcium in the blood which in turn can affect the conduction of nerve impulses and the contraction of muscles. The end result or effect is that the person then experiences painful tingling in the hands and toes, which can then become flexed and contracted in a cramped posture. This is sometimes called tetany (being quite different from the infection called tetanus). The lack of carbon dioxide also produces a feeling of light-headedness or dizziness, and the whole episode may then be confused with a seizure. Treatment is simple and dramatically effective. A paper or, if no paper bag is available, a small plastic bag is placed (temporarily!) over the patient's nose and mouth, so that she re-breathes her own expired air, which is rich in carbon dioxide. This then resets the body chemistry and the person usually rapidly recovers. This is what happens when someone is described as having a panic attack.

Simulated seizures also known as non-epileptic attack disorder (NEAD) or psychogenic, non-epileptic seizures (PNES)

These are often called 'simulated' seizures—because they may look like an epileptic seizure. It might seem strange that anyone would want to behave or pretend that they are having an epileptic seizure, but in many hospital consultants' experience this is one of the more common differential diagnoses that must be considered. The great majority of such patients have some knowledge of epilepsy; either they have seen a relative with seizures, or more commonly they have had some real (true) seizures themselves. Unless the real (true) and suspect (simulated or non-real) attacks are both seen by an expert, it may be impossible to sort out exactly what is happening. A doctor may be mistaken and deceived into giving more and more anti-epileptic drugs for seizures which he believes to be out of control. Conversely, if he sees one seizure or fit which he is quite sure is not epileptic, he may well wrongly believe all of them are feigned.

The most common type of seizure which is simulated or mimed is a tonic–clonic seizure. However, other seizures may also be simulated, including absence and focal seizures.

The points which distinguish a true and simulated seizure are the character of the convulsions, which are often not imitated very well. These include the following features:

- Most non-epileptic seizures occur when there are many people around and these seizures appear to intensify when someone tries to intervene.

- The eyes are usually open during a real or true tonic–clonic seizure but are shut during a non-real seizure. During a simulated or non-real seizure, if someone tries to open the person's eyes, they are shut even tighter!

- The facial jerking and excessive salivation are very difficult to mimic in a simulated or non-epileptic tonic–clonic seizure.

- It is very uncommon for a person to deliberately bite their tongue in a simulated or non-epileptic (non-real) tonic–clonic seizure.

- A non-epileptic tonic–clonic seizure starts and ends very abruptly, and may happen repeatedly over many minutes. In contrast, a genuine tonic–clonic seizure starts and ends gradually and the person will usually only have one seizure.

- The recovery from a real tonic–clonic seizure usually takes some time, often at least one half to an hour or more, whilst recovery from a non-real seizure can be immediate or quite rapid, occurring within 5 or 10 minutes.

- A normal EEG recorded during a generalized tonic–clonic 'seizure' is virtually incontrovertible evidence of simulation. However, the EEG record may be so technically affected and even spoiled by the patient's thrashing around that interpretation may be difficult. Combined video and EEG recording with the person as an inpatient (video-EEG telemetry) may sometimes have to be undertaken in the more difficult-to-diagnose situations.

Urinary incontinence does not always distinguish between true and simulated seizures as this can sometimes be simulated—and this feature is far more commonly seen in adults rather than in children.

Psychiatrists seem to make a distinction between simulation of disease due to conscious malingering, for example, a man keen to avoid family or work responsibilities (including in the past, conscription into the army); and unconscious hysteria, in which it is alleged the simulation is the product of the unconscious mind. Sometimes the reason is because the person wants help for a problem but is either not able to ask, or is afraid to ask for it. This may be because they are being bullied or are being subject to physical or sexual abuse. The reward in simulating seizures usually is then to gain this attention, and so obtain help. Rather than lay blame, doctors should regard these events as an indication that patients cannot cope with their life problems, try and identify the problems that are causing the simulated seizures and then help them find a solution. Blaming someone or accusing them of wasting the doctors' time is unhelpful and may actually make the situation far worse, and in the long term, much more difficult to help the person. However, it is often the case that individuals will have a combination of both epileptic seizures and psychogenic, non-epileptic seizures—and this does make their treatment more difficult.

Miscellaneous

Finally, seizures may occur in a number of other, systemic illnesses or situations including:

- after a sudden blow to the head called a concussive convulsion. This can occur when there has been a sudden bang or injury to the head, as when falling off a horse or when there is a collision of heads during a rugby or football match. Almost immediately or within no more than a second or two, the person will start jerking or 'convulsing' and this may last for about a minute. The jerking is not the same as the jerking that occurs in a tonic–clonic seizure. Although a concussive convulsion follows an injury it is not quite the same thing as a reflex anoxic seizure which has been discussed earlier in this chapter.

- hypoglycaemia (low blood sugar; this may occur in treated diabetes mellitus if too much insulin is given)

- hypocalcaemia (low blood calcium; this is particularly likely to occur in infants and young children and in strict vegetarians)

- renal (kidney), hepatic (liver) and respiratory (lung) failure

- meningitis and encephalitis

- alcohol abuse and its withdrawal

- inborn errors of body metabolism (Chapter 3).

Finally, the potential effects of prescription or illicit (including recreational) drugs in precipitating seizures must always be considered; there are many types of recreational drugs but the more common ones include ecstasy, heroin and cannabis.

5

Tests in epilepsy

→ Key points

- Epilepsy is a clinical diagnosis and is made by taking a very detailed history or account of a person's clinical events.

- Epilepsy should not be diagnosed on the results of any tests without evidence that the person is actually having epileptic seizures.

- There is no single test that can always make or rule out a diagnosis of epilepsy.

- Every child and most adults who have had a diagnosis of epilepsy made on the basis of a detailed and accurate history, should have an electroencephalogram (EEG).

- The EEG can be very helpful in identifying a particular epilepsy syndrome and as a guide for which anti-epileptic drug may be useful in treating a person's seizures.

- Brain scans using magnetic resonance imaging (MRI) or computerized tomography (CT) are important in helping to find a cause for a person's epilepsy.

- Most but not all people with focal (partial) seizures will need to have a brain scan.

- Very few people with generalized seizures will need to have a brain scan.

- Other tests, such as blood and urine tests, are not particularly helpful in most patients who have epilepsy.

The previous chapter has made it clear that epilepsy is a clinical diagnosis based on a full, accurate and detailed description of events. There is no single test which can always make, or exclude, a diagnosis of epilepsy. Moreover, as also explained in earlier chapters, epilepsy is not a single condition. There are many different types of epilepsy and epilepsy syndromes, and there are many different causes of epilepsy. Tests or investigations may be useful to:

◆ add weight to, or support the clinical diagnosis of epilepsy

◆ help classify the type of epileptic seizure and epilepsy syndrome. This is important in predicting the likely outcome of the epilepsy in a given individual, and the treatment that should be used

◆ help detect or find a cause for the epilepsy

◆ as has been shown in Table 3.2 (Chapter 3), no obvious cause will be found in one half to about two-thirds of children and adults with epilepsy

◆ there is a greater chance of finding a cause in people with focal (partial), rather than generalized seizures

◆ the main investigations which may be used in epilepsy are the electro-encephalogram (EEG) and brain imaging techniques, most commonly magnetic resonance imaging (MRI) and computerized tomography (CT) scanning. Other investigations such as blood tests, lumbar puncture (spinal tap), X-rays or tissue biopsy are much less commonly undertaken. These tests will be undertaken in individuals who usually have additional medical problems or if their epilepsy worsens over a period of time.

Electroencephalography (EEG)

The EEG is the principal investigation used in epilepsy. Most, if not all, patients with epilepsy will have an EEG performed, usually after a clinical diagnosis has been made, and ideally before treatment is started. The EEG detects the brain's electrical activity by sensitive sensors called electrodes which are placed on the scalp; these electrodes detect the normal and abnormal electrical activity of the nerve cells within the brain. Most routine EEGs are recorded with the child or adult awake, but EEGs may be arranged after deprivation of sleep or during sleep (natural sleep or sleep induced by drugs).

All hospitals with neurological or neurosurgical departments and some larger, non-specialized hospitals will have facilities for recording a routine EEG. The procedure is simple and painless and a routine EEG takes only about 20–30 minutes to complete. The EEG only detects and records the brain's activity;

at no time is there any electrical discharge passing from the equipment to the patient. The EEG should not be confused with electroconvulsive therapy or ECT, which is used to treat depressive illnesses, and has nothing to do with epilepsy.

The recording technician (called a clinical physiologist) first measures the patient's head for correct placement of the electrodes, which are then placed according to an international system based on the patient's head size and on measurements taken from the bridge of the nose, and the bony protuberance at the back of the head (called the occiput). Silver electrodes are fastened to the head with a sticky and rather pungent (smelly) substance called collodion. Alternatively, the electrodes are gauze pads moistened with a salt solution and secured over the head with a rubber cap. Sometimes the patient's scalp is gently rubbed beneath the electrodes to reduce the electrical resistance of the skin which improves the recording. For a routine EEG, 12 electrodes are used in small infants, 20 in older children and adults. Wires from each electrode are then connected to a junction box (head-box), connected in turn to the amplifiers of the EEG machine by a cable. After amplification, the EEG machine records the signals. In the past this was on tape or disc, or directly by ink-jets, pens, or laser on to paper which moves at constant speed, usually 3 cm/second. However, the vast majority of EEG recording is now paperless and recorded digitally, and can be read directly from a computer screen. It is this pattern of digital recording on the computer screen (or, rarely, on paper), that is known as 'the EEG' and which is examined and analysed by doctors (Figure 5.1). One of the many advantages of digital EEG recordings is that the pattern of how the electrodes are placed on the scalp, called the montage, can be rapidly changed between different montages to try and more accurately identify where there may be a specific abnormality. This is particularly useful if the patient has focal or partial seizures.

During an EEG the child or adult is asked to lie quite still. This is because movement of any part of the body may obscure, or make it difficult to detect the electrical activity of the brain. This movement activity is called artefact. Any movement, including chewing or sucking, or a parent gently patting a child's back or bouncing them up and down on their knee to comfort them may produce an artefact that may not just obscure the brain's electrical activity but might even sometimes appear very similar to epileptic activity on the EEG.

The EEG physiologist during the course of the recording will also ask the patient to open and close their eyes (to look for normal patterns of activity which vary according to whether the eyes are opened or not), to over-breathe for 3 or 4 minutes, and to look at a flashing light. Over-breathing (which is

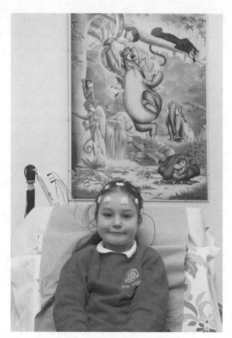

Figure 5.1 A child having a routine EEG recorded.

called hyperventilation) and the flashing-light test (called intermittent photic stimulation) are useful ways of activating or provoking abnormal electrical activity from the brain, and are often important in helping to decide what type of seizure or what type of epilepsy syndrome a person has (Chapter 2).

◆ Hyperventilation is very effective in inducing one or more typical absence seizures in a child with the epilepsy syndrome of childhood-onset absence epilepsy. In fact, if the child hyperventilates very well for 3 or 4 minutes and does not have an absence seizure, then it is very unlikely that they have childhood-onset absence epilepsy. Hyperventilation may also induce atypical absences in some of the other absence epilepsy syndromes, including absence with myoclonus. Hyperventilation is not particularly helpful in adults and rarely induces any type of seizure, including an absence seizure.

◆ Intermittent photic stimulation uses a light, called a *stroboscope*, placed about 6 to 9 inches from the patient's eyes, which flashes at different frequencies. This varies from 1 flash per second up to about 50 flashes per second. The most common type of photosensitivity occurs when the light flashes at about 14–30 flashes per second. This type of photosensitivity is seen in at least 50 per cent of individuals with juvenile myoclonic epilepsy, one of the idiopathic or primary generalized epilepsy syndromes. A much rarer type of photosensitivity is seen when the light flashes at 1 flash per second and is seen in young children with a rare and progressive type of epilepsy and severe learning difficulties, called late infantile Batten's disease. In fact, the type of photosensitivity in this condition may provide the first clue that this might be the underlying diagnosis.

The appearance of the EEG is dependent upon the age of a patient. This is because the brain is developing and maturing rapidly, particularly from birth to 8 or 10 years of age. Generally speaking, a normal adult EEG pattern (Figure 5.2) is reached by the age of 10-12 years and there is then little change until the age of 60 or 70 years. Doctors who analyse EEGs must have appropriate training and know about the EEG patterns (normal and abnormal) in babies (including babies who are born prematurely), infants and children, as well as in adults.

The hallmark or typical EEG finding in a patient with epilepsy between seizures, called the inter-ictal EEG, is a 'spike' or 'spike and slow wave' or 'sharp wave'. A spike is a sudden change in voltage that shows up against the background activities. Sometimes two or more spikes may occur together, and the EEG appearance of this is called *polyspikes* ('poly' meaning many). Spikes and slow waves and sharp waves are often referred to as epileptiform or epileptic activity. Examples of focal and generalized EEG abnormalities are shown in Figures 5.3 and 5.4. An example of a very abnormal EEG seen in infants with West syndrome (Chapter 2) is shown in Figure 5.6. However, even in patients who have epilepsy these abnormalities are not always seen, and this is why the EEG must not be relied upon to make or exclude a diagnosis of epilepsy. The first 20 minutes of an EEG recording of an adult who has had an undoubted tonic–clonic seizure will be normal in 40–50 per cent of cases. Conversely, the EEG will be abnormal, including showing epileptiform activity, in 5–10 per cent of school-age children who have never had—and who never will have—any type of epileptic seizure.

For most people with epilepsy, a routine (20–30 minute) EEG is the only necessary test. However, this is only a short period to record the brain's electrical activity. This, together with the fact that the EEG is being undertaken in an artificial environment (whether the patient is a child or an adult), means that it is very unlikely that a clinical attack or seizure will occur in this time. The only exceptions to this are if the child has childhood-onset absence epilepsy or the patient is photosensitive when they may have a brief myoclonic (jerk) seizure whilst they are undergoing intermittent photic stimulation. If more

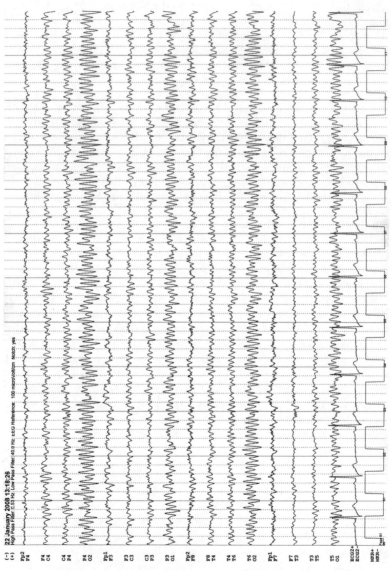

Figure 5.2 A normal EEG pattern. This pattern is seen from mid-childhood (age 10–12 years) until late adult life (60+ years).

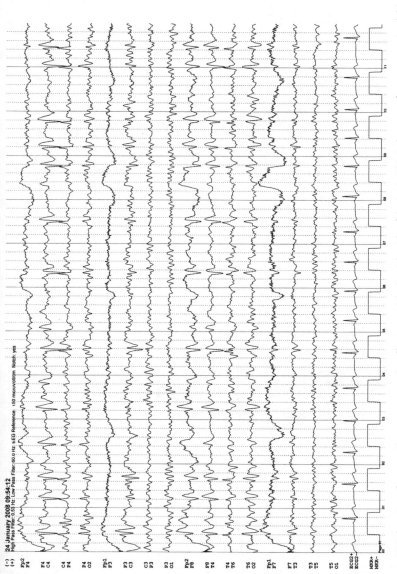

Figure 5.3 EEG showing a frequent sharp wave or spike affecting mainly the right side of the brain. This is the type of pattern seen in children and adults with a focal (partial) epilepsy. This particular individual is a 10-year-old child with the common epilepsy syndrome that occurs in children called benign partial epilepsy with centro-temporal spikes.

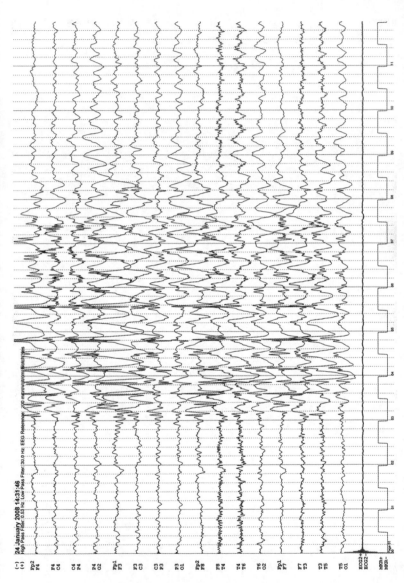

Figure 5.4 EEG of a young child showing a 5 to 6 second burst of rhythmic generalized spike and slow wave activity which was associated with a brief absence seizure. The child is a 7-year-old girl with childhood-onset absence epilepsy. This is an example of primary or idiopathic generalized epilepsy.

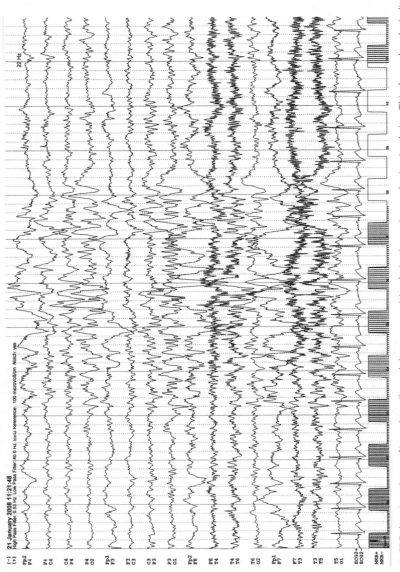

Figure 5.5 EEG showing a burst of irregular spike and slow wave activity during intermittent photic stimulation. This shows that the individual is photosensitive. The patient is a 16-year-old with another type of primary or idiopathic generalized epilepsy, called juvenile myoclonic epilepsy.

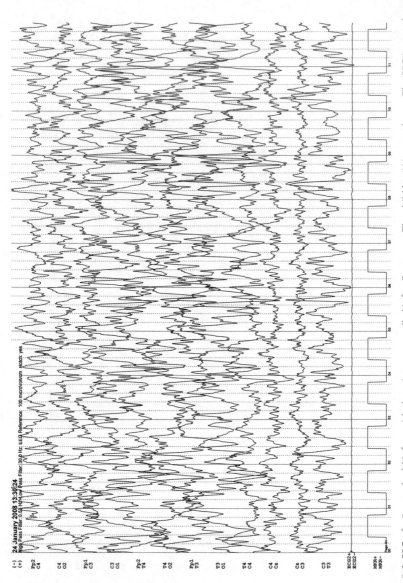

Figure 5.6 EEG of a 7-month old infant with the seizure type called infantile spasms. The child has West syndrome. The EEG is very abnormal with no normal electrical activity from the brain; this pattern is called hypsarrhythmia.

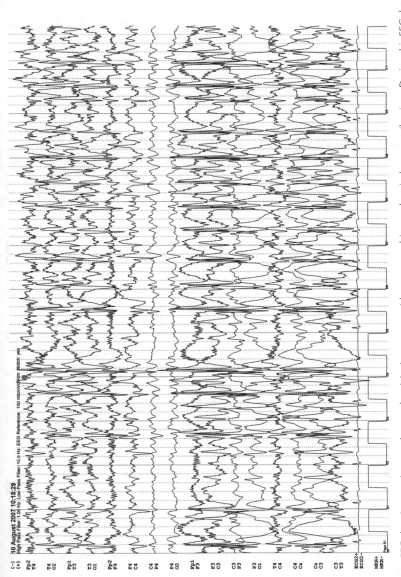

Figure 5.7 EEG showing continuous abnormal activity in a person with non-convulsive or electrical status epilepticus. During this EEG the child was only partly responsive and kept having little jerks (myoclonic seizures) and brief absences. The child has the epilepsy syndrome called severe myoclonic epilepsy of infancy (Dravet syndrome).

information is required, then other types or systems of EEG recording may be performed.

◆ *EEG after deprivation of sleep*: In this situation a patient is asked to make sure they get only 4–5 hours sleep for two consecutive nights. This encourages the occurrence of seizure discharges. Deprivation of sleep may also lead the patient to nap or to sleep during the recording, and again this encourages the appearance of abnormal EEG discharge. It may also lower the threshold for the person to actually have a seizure.

◆ *Drug-induced sleeping EEG*: A small dose of a sedative drug or a drug called melatonin may encourage the patient to fall asleep during the recording, and again drowsiness and sleep may show abnormalities which may not be present whilst awake.

◆ *Ambulatory EEG monitoring*: This is a technique of recording an EEG for not just 20 or 30 minutes but for up to 24 or even 48 hours, or longer. The electrodes (six, eight or twelve, occasionally more) are wired up to a small tape recorder (like a Walkman cassette player) which is strapped to the waist. After this, the child or adult can leave the EEG department, go home and carry on their normal activities, and then return to the EEG department after 24 hours to have the tape analysed or the tape replaced. This procedure is more likely, by the length of the recording and the fact that the individual is able to be in their usual environment, to pick up abnormal electrical activity and even capture one or more of their usual seizures. The tape can be analysed in a special fast-pace display unit, so the doctor does not have to sit watching the EEG for 24-48 hours!

◆ *Depth electrodes*: On rare occasions, special depth electrodes are used. These are fine wires inserted under sterile conditions into areas of the brain thought possibly to be the site of origin of seizure discharge. Areas of the brain implanted with these electrodes are usually the temporal lobes. This is an important test in those patients who are being considered for surgical treatment of their epilepsy (Chapter 6).

◆ *Grid or mat electrodes*: These electrodes are used when considering a surgical treatment for the patient's epilepsy. Rather than a single, needle-like electrode (as in recording a depth EEG described above), these are arranged in a rectangular or square mat or grid which may contain 32, 64 or even more flat electrodes, like the ones used for a routine scalp EEG. The skull is opened and the mat or grid is placed directly on the surface of the brain, over where it is thought the abnormal nerve cells are located. One or two wires are attached to the mat or grid and then the skull is closed and the wires are attached to the EEG machine. Recording can continue for as long as it takes for the patient to have some of their usual seizures. This is very useful in locating precisely where within the cerebral cortex the seizures may be coming from. This technique is often used in patients with focal seizures arising from either the frontal or temporal lobes. The term for both depth and mat or grid EEG recording is 'invasive EEG monitoring or recording' and can only be undertaken in very specialized epilepsy centres. Both techniques are only used when there is a sure possibility that a surgical procedure might be possible to treat a person's epilepsy.

◆ *Video-telemetry*: This is another way of obtaining an EEG over a longer period of time. In this technique the patient has to stay in a room in the hospital for 24 hours or longer. At the same time as the electrical activity is recorded on the EEG, a video camera records the activities of the patient (Figure 5.7). In this way, it is possible to replay repeatedly both simultaneous video and closed circuit television (CCTV) and EEG recordings, and observe the pattern of the EEG during a seizure or attack. This provides valuable information on the type of epileptic seizure and from where within the brain the seizure may be starting. If no abnormalities are seen on the EEG during a seizure or an attack, then this strongly suggests that the seizures or attacks are not epileptic. The exception to this is if the seizures are coming from deep within one of the frontal lobes. Video-telemetry is really only of practical benefit if the patient is having frequent attacks, as it is otherwise impractical to keep the patient in hospital attached to expensive equipment on the remote chance that a seizure may occur. Sometimes a patient's anti-epileptic medication is reduced before they are admitted to increase the chance of recording the person's usual seizures during the video-EEG telemetry. This technique can be undertaken with surface electrodes (as in Figure 5.8) or with depth, mat or grid electrodes.

◆ Finally, there is a new EEG technique, called magnetoelectro-encephalography (MEG), which is being developed in a few epilepsy centres, and mainly for research. Sometimes, MEG is also used with neuro-imaging to help find a focus for a person's epilepsy. MEG is therefore most likely to be helpful in planning a surgical treatment for a person's epilepsy. It is unclear as to whether MEG will ever be used as a routine EEG test in most patients with epilepsy or not. Probably not.

How sensitive is the EEG?

The EEG is often thought to be able either to prove, or to exclude a diagnosis of epilepsy, but this is rarely possible. A single, routine EEG is likely to show

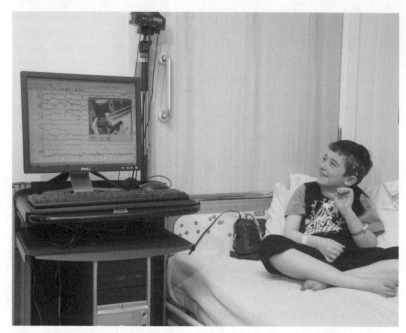

Figure 5.8 A child having a video-EEG telemetry recording. At the same time as the brain's electrical activity is being recorded, continuous closed-circuit TV (CCTV) records the child's behaviour and movements. This means that when the child has a seizure, it is possible to correlate precisely their movements and behaviour during the seizure with what is happening electrically in the brain.

any abnormal (and therefore helpful) activity in only about half of those who have had a tonic–clonic seizure. If additional and/or longer duration EEGs are done, particularly after sleep-deprivation, the yield and chance of finding abnormalities increases. It must therefore be clearly understood that the EEG does not necessarily prove, nor disprove the diagnosis of epilepsy. There are really only three important exceptions to this important rule and these are as follows:

- in childhood-onset absence epilepsy; the EEG, and particularly if the child performed hyperventilation well, will record a typical absence in over 95 per cent of children; conversely, if the EEG is normal then it is very unlikely that the child has this epilepsy syndrome

- in children thought to have infantile spasms (West syndrome, Chapter 2), a sleeping EEG will always show hypsarrhythmia; if a sleeping EEG does not show hypsarrhythmia, then the child will not have West syndrome

- in a person with a type of epilepsy called non-convulsive status epilepticus (Chapter 2). This may present with bizarre or confused behaviour with semi-purposeful, almost automatic movements. It may be difficult to decide whether this behaviour is epilepsy, but if it is, the EEG is usually very helpful in making the diagnosis.

> The most important point is that the EEG alone should not be used to either confirm (make) or exclude (rule out) a diagnosis of epilepsy.

The EEG is also not a good guide to either assess the severity or the prognosis, also called the outcome, of epilepsy. There are two types of epilepsy, or epilepsy syndromes, in which the EEG is particularly useful—and both of these have already been mentioned above. One is childhood-onset absence epilepsy where the frequent seizures may be so brief and subtle that some time may elapse before they are recognized. In children with typical absences, the EEG almost always shows a seizure discharge, which nearly always is induced by hyperventilation, and even more easily after deprivation of sleep. The second is West syndrome, in which the seizure type is infantile spasms.

It is only occasionally necessary to repeat the EEG in a patient with epilepsy. However, there are some exceptions to this general rule. Further EEGs may be helpful if treatment is not as effective as expected, or if, after a period of good seizure control, a patient's seizures become more frequent. Some doctors recommend that an EEG should be repeated before a patient comes off treatment with anti-epileptic drugs, but there is not much evidence that this helps reach a decision.

Table 3.2 shows that for nearly two-thirds of cases a cause of epilepsy is not found. The EEG is usually not helpful in identifying a cause. Occasionally, however, the EEG may show a pattern that is very characteristic of a specific cause of the epilepsy. Examples of these causes include a condition called sub-acute sclerosing panencephalitis (SSPE) which is related to measles infection, particularly in those children who have not been immunized (vaccinated) against measles or who had measles under two years of age. Another is a condition called late infantile Batten's disease. Occasionally, there may be a marked difference in the electrical activity between the two sides of the brain, where a slow wave discharge or sharp and slow wave discharge is seen only in one half of the brain, or in one particular part (lobe) of the brain. This could suggest the presence of a structural abnormality as the cause of the patient's epilepsy—such as an area of abnormal brain development (the technical term for this is cerebral dysgenesis or cortical dysplasia), result of scarring (such as following meningitis) or, particularly in teenagers and adults, a brain tumour. However, structural abnormalities are best investigated by imaging techniques (brain scans). These are, after the EEG, the most commonly used type of investigation in epilepsy.

Brain imaging investigations

The EEG is a functional investigation, recording the brain's function through normal and abnormal electrical activity. Most imaging procedures or brain scans provide information about the brain's structure, and can reveal normal and abnormal anatomy. Most, if not all, patients who have epilepsy need to have at least one EEG, but less than 1 in 5 or 1 in 6 patients need to have an imaging investigation.

Two types of imaging techniques are currently available in the developed world; these are the computerized tomography (CT) brain scan and magnetic resonance imaging (MRI). More sophisticated imaging techniques have also become available over the past decade or so which are the more functional types of brain imaging. These include functional MRI (known as fMRI), SPECT (single photon emission computerized tomography) and PET (positron emission tomography). The precise role of these three latter imaging techniques in the investigation and treatment of the epilepsies has yet to be decided.

The CT scan

This is an abbreviation for either computerized axial tomography (CAT) or computerized tomography (CT) scan. The technique was developed in the 1970s and is a type of X-ray investigation. Tomography is a word dating from earlier X-ray techniques. The patient lies still on a table whilst a rotating X-ray machine takes two-dimensional pictures of the head from many different angles or positions (see Figure 5.9). The information is then processed by a computer to produce pictures (or images) at different levels of the brain. Examples of a normal and abnormal CT scan are shown in Figures 5.10 and 5.11. The test is safe, and other than keeping the head still, there are no particular precautions to be taken. However, it does involve some irradiation. Children may sometimes have to be given a sedative drug or short general anaesthetic so that they can keep still for the scan. The test used to take up to 20 minutes but more state-of-the-art scanners take just 30–60 seconds. If an area of interest (possible

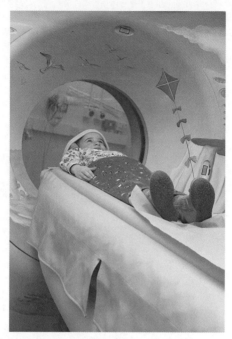

Figure 5.9 Child having a computerized tomography (CT) brain scan. These days a CT scan can be done in just 30–60 seconds.

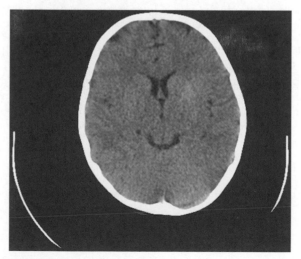

Figure 5.10 Normal CT brain scan.

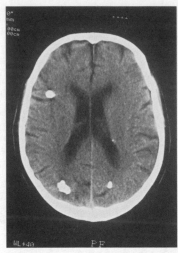

Figure 5.11 An abnormal CT head scan in an 11-year old child showing areas of calcification (the bright white 'spots') and abnormal brain development. This child has the condition called tuberous sclerosis which was first seen at 8 months of age with infantile spasms. Many years later, the child has poorly controlled focal (partial) seizures.

abnormality) is seen on the initial images, some contrast (special dye) is injected into a vein in the hand or arm and then the scan repeated. The dye may enhance contrast in the area of interest and may provide further useful information as to the nature or cause of the possible abnormality.

When CT scanning was first introduced many years ago, it proved to be very useful in detecting structural abnormalities within the brain, such as strokes, infections, tumours, and major congenital malformations which may cause epilepsy. However, only 20–25 per cent of patients with epilepsy referred to special centres will have an abnormal CT scan. Abnormalities on the CT scan in patients who have epilepsy are more likely to be found in the following situations:

- patients whose seizures affect only one side of the body;

- patients whose EEG shows a persistent slow wave abnormality on one side of the brain;

- when epilepsy starts in newborn babies and continues;

- when epilepsy starts in later life; and

◆ if the patient has abnormal findings on neurological examination, for example, mild weakness down one side of the body, many birthmarks (white or coffee-coloured marks in the skin) or changes in the muscle stretch reflexes.

If the result of the CT scan is not always clear and further information is needed, then the person should also have an MRI scan. In view of this, an MRI scan is now nearly always preferred to a CT scan when doing brain scans in people with epilepsy.

The MR scan (MRI)

MRI (magnetic resonance imaging) or nuclear magnetic resonance (NMR), has nothing to do with radiation or X-rays, but records energy given out by atoms as they change their orientation after a brief magnetic pulse. The pictures or images produced have the same general appearance as CT scans, because the information processed by the computer is much the same (Figures 5.12 and 5.13). However, the images produced by an MRI scan are much clearer and far more detailed than a CT scan. Because of this, MRI has now replaced CT as the preferred imaging method when investigating patients with epilepsy. Again, it is necessary for the patient to lie still while the images are being taken. Because an MRI scan takes between 20 and 30 minutes (sometimes longer) to complete, it is actually more important for the person to lie very still.

The procedure is noisier than CT scanning and may, in some patients, produce a claustrophobic feeling, as the individual is partly enclosed in what looks like a small tunnel. Occasionally some contrast dye, called gadolinium, is injected into a vein, as in CT scanning, and then the scan repeated to demonstrate some additional details. Children may find the procedure more uncomfortable than having a CT scan and because of this, more often need to have a brief general anaesthetic. MRI gives a much clearer picture of those areas of the brain (the temporal lobes) which are most often responsible for intractable focal epilepsy (Figure 5.15, p. 94), and so patients who are considered possibly to be suitable for surgery will certainly need an MRI. MRI is also useful for children in whom the epilepsy is thought to be due to a congenital malformation of the brain because it will show up areas of cortical dysplasia which are often missed on a CT scan. MRI costs significantly more than CT but the extra cost is more than justified because of its advantages over CT.

There is rarely any justification for routinely repeating a CT or MRI brain scan. However, if something suspicious is seen on a CT scan, then an MRI scan should always be undertaken to confirm any abnormality, particularly if surgery for the epilepsy is being considered. In fact, as has been stated earlier

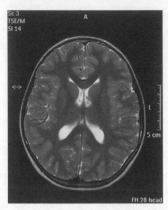

Figure 5.12 Normal MRI scan; an MRI of a person's brain can normally be done in 20–30 minutes.

in this chapter, MRI has largely replaced CT as the preferred, and therefore, the first, imaging technique. If a person's epilepsy deteriorates, or the patient develops new symptoms such as weakness of a limb or develops new neurological signs, then it is essential to investigate the patient again and this will usually be with an MRI rather than a CT scan. This is because sometimes, even if there is a structural abnormality causing the epilepsy, this might

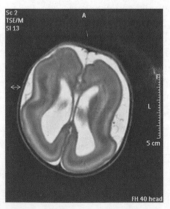

Figure 5.13 An abnormal MRI scan in a 1-year-old child with daily myoclonic and tonic seizures and severe developmental delay. The surface of the brain is very smooth. This is called lissencephaly (which means 'smooth brain').

not have been seen on a first scan and may only be seen on a second scan undertaken a year or more later.

Other imaging techniques

Over the past few years, new imaging techniques have become available and are particularly useful when considering a surgical procedure to treat the epilepsy. These are known as functional imaging techniques because in addition to showing some structures in the brain they also show how the brain is functioning. The three most commonly used functional imaging techniques include:

◆ functional MRI (abbreviated to fMRI)

◆ SPECT scanning (which stands for single photon emission computed tomography)

◆ PET scanning (which stands for positron emission tomography).

Functional MRI: This is a way at looking at small and specific areas of the brain that are activated when someone does or says something. During these

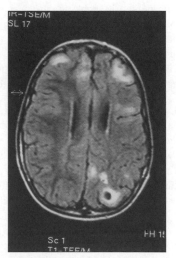

Figure 5.14 An abnormal MRI scan in a 15-year-old with tuberous sclerosis—the same condition, but in a different person, seen in Figure 5.11.

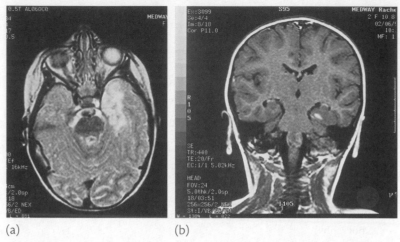

(a)   (b)

Figure 5.15 Two different views of an abnormal MRI scan in a 14-year-old with frequent focal (partial) seizures and short-term memory difficulties. In (a), the abnormal white area in the left temporal lobe is caused by a developmental abnormality called a hamartoma. This is also seen in (b) but in addition, part of the temporal lobe is abnormally large.

movements or when the person is speaking, the nerve cells and their blood supply in these regions are activated and can be shown up on an MRI scan. This technique is important in mapping parts of the brain that are likely to be involved in very important in key activities such as speaking, memory, movement, and some learning tasks. Functional MRI is becoming increasingly important in preparing individuals for surgery to treat their epilepsy.

SPECT and PET: Both SPECT and PET use a technique which involves injecting a marker (called a radioactive tracer) into the patient. SPECT is much cheaper and much simpler to undertake but may not always produce as good images as PET. With SPECT, an example of one such tracer is 99mTc-hexamethylpropyleneamineoxime. With PET, the tracer is a glucose solution (the tracer is called 18F-2-deoxyglucose) or, less commonly, breathing oxygen (the tracer is called 15O-labelled water). The technetium (Tc), glucose or oxygen is taken up and metabolized by different parts of the brain at different rates. The marker atoms (tracers) attached to the technetium (99mTc), oxygen (15O) or glucose (18F) allow images to be obtained which may show an area or areas of the brain which take up a lot of oxygen and glucose during a seizure, and which could be an epileptic focus; these are called areas of hyperperfusion. Between seizures, the same areas are relatively silent; these are called areas of hypoperfusion. Both SPECT and PET are mainly used in research but also in specialist epilepsy centres which carry out detailed and sophisticated surgical techniques in patients with epilepsy and other neurological conditions, including movement disorders, Parkinson's disease and dystonia.

It is almost certain that fMRI and SPECT scanning, but probably not PET scanning, will become more routinely available over the next few years. It is also very likely that other imaging techniques will be developed in the next few years.

Cerebral angiography

Another technique, cerebral angiography, is still occasionally used in some patients with epilepsy where the cause is thought to be due to an abnormal collection of blood vessels in the brain (either an arterio-venous malformation or cavernous haemangioma). In this technique, an iodine-containing solution which is opaque to X-rays is injected directly into one or the other carotid artery (in the neck), or through a catheter introduced into the brachial (elbow) or femoral (groin) arteries and passed into the region of the carotid artery. Immediately after the injection, a series of X-ray pictures are taken which outline the arteries and veins containing the iodine solution. This technique precisely identifies any abnormal blood vessels and may be extremely valuable if surgery is being considered on an arterio-venous malformation or haemangioma or tumour, and particularly, if any of these abnormalities are located deep within the brain. Although advances in MRI mean that the circulation can usually be imaged by special pulse techniques and image processing software in a technique called MRA (magnetic resonance angiography), it is unlikely that this will replace conventional cerebral angiography in most situations.

Before the development of CT scanning, simple skull X-rays or air-encephalograms (in which the structure of the brain was outlined by injected air administered by a lumbar puncture or spinal tap) were the only techniques available to look at the brain. These have been completely superseded by MRI and CT scans.

Other tests

Blood and urine tests are rarely helpful in patients with epilepsy. However, some blood tests may be useful, particularly in the early days or weeks of life, when chemical abnormalities, such as low blood levels of glucose (called hypoglycaemia), calcium (called hypocalcaemia) or, rarely, magnesium (called hypomagnesaemia) may cause seizures. These biochemical abnormalities usually cause frequent seizures and usually of the myoclonic, clonic and tonic–clonic type (Chapter 2).

Genetic tests may also be carried out on blood samples, looking for an abnormality in the patient's chromosomes (as in the condition called ring chromosome 20) or DNA (as in severe myoclonic epilepsy of infancy [Dravet syndrome] and conditions such as tuberous sclerosis, Angelman and Rett syndrome). These genetic tests are helpful in diagnosing a specific cause of the epilepsy. They are also helpful in genetic counselling, and particularly, in predicting how likely it is to recur within other family members and other children. Almost certainly, future advances in genetics will enable doctors to find out much more about why epilepsy occurs and to identify specific causes of epilepsy. Other, more sophisticated blood tests may also need to be carried out, depending on the overall clinical situation.

A lumbar puncture (also called a spinal tap), may be carried out if an infection such as meningitis or encephalitis is suspected to be causing epileptic seizures (Chapter 2). Sometimes, and particularly in children, the fluid obtained from the lumbar puncture, called the cerebrospinal fluid or CSF, may reveal chemical or metabolic abnormalities that may be responsible for the child's epilepsy. Children with a metabolic disorder, and particularly one called a mitochondrial disorder, usually have other problems also, including developmental delay, learning or visual difficulties or poor growth, including poor head growth. Analysis of the CSF may also be able to diagnose an infection such as meningitis or encephalitis which often presents with seizures in babies and children.

Occasionally, removal of tissues (biopsy) for microscopic analysis may be helpful in finding out rare causes of epilepsy; the tissues which are biopsied include skin or rectum (as these contain accessible nerve cells) or muscle. The diseases which are being tested for are rare and usually have manifestations other than seizures alone.

Sometimes, it may be necessary to biopsy the brain if an abnormality is found on the MRI brain scan and the nature or cause of this abnormality is not known. The biopsy may be important in diagnosing:

♦ a brain tumour

♦ an area of abnormal brain development (called cortical dysplasia)

♦ an area of chronic inflammation such as in Rasmussen's syndrome.

Summary

In summary, all patients in whom epilepsy is diagnosed on the basis of a detailed and accurate history should have an EEG to help diagnose the type of epilepsy syndrome and provide guidance on the most appropriate anti-epileptic medication. The much more expensive tape-recorded EEGs and video monitoring of seizures do undoubtedly help discriminate between different types of seizures, and between real and simulated attacks. Most, but not necessarily all, people with a focal or partial epilepsy should have a brain scan and this should be an MRI scan. Otherwise, laboratory investigation of seizures has a limited value.

The neurologist will decide on the most relevant investigations that should be undertaken and discuss this with their patients.

The technical aspects of the neurological consultation—the detailed history, the differential diagnosis, the examination, any necessary investigation, and prescription of anti-epileptic drug—take comparatively little time. The most important component or part of the initial consultation with the patient (or if the patient is a young child, with their parents), is taking a full and detailed history to ensure that the diagnosis of epilepsy is secure. The other, next most important part of the consultation should be spent, in our view, in exploring the person's (or parents', or both) attitudes and knowledge about epilepsy, and the effect that epilepsy may have on their life, so that practical advice and support can be given. This usually has to take two or more consultations, and involve the input and skills of an epilepsy nurse specialist. How much of ongoing support should be provided by the neurologist and the epilepsy nurse specialist and how much by the family doctor depends upon the personalities of the doctors and the patient, as well as upon the available time. What is disastrous for the patient is if each doctor assumes that the other is coping with these aspects. This is discussed in far more detail in Chapters 6 and 8.

6

The treatment of epilepsy

> **Key points**
>
> - A thorough assessment of the seizure type and cause should be made before considering anti-epileptic drug treatment.
>
> - After a first seizure, anti-epileptic drug treatment reduces the risk of a second seizure from around 40 per cent to 30 per cent over 2 years but may be associated with adverse effects such that there is no clear advantage from either alternative.
>
> - There are many anti-epileptic drugs to choose from.
>
> - Some drugs are more effective for certain types of epilepsy than others, and a decision as to which drug to start requires a thorough discussion of likely benefits and side-effects of the possible treatments.
>
> - Anti-epileptic drugs can cause abnormality in the developing child (foetus) with around 5 per cent having a major malformation such as spina bifida. This should be discussed with all young women.
>
> - Brain surgery may be a treatment option for some patients whose seizures are not controlled by anti-epileptic drugs, particularly those with temporal lobe epilepsy.

The first step is to identify whether seizures have occurred, which requires the doctor to take a careful history and, where necessary, organize investigations such as an EEG and/or a brain scan (CT or MRI) . It is important to differentiate seizures from other causes of funny turn or collapse. For example, people who faint may have brief stiffness and jerking of their limbs which can be mistaken for an epileptic seizure, whilst in children there are other sort of attacks which might be misdiagnosed as seizures. Where seizures have occurred, the doctor will need to try and identify the type or types of seizures, their cause, and the type of epilepsy (epilepsy syndrome, see Chapter 2), as these, along with other factors, will influence the type of treatment that is recommended. This chapter focuses mainly upon drug treatments and there are two terms usually applied to drug treatments for epilepsy—anti-epileptic drugs and anti-convulsants. In this chapter we will refer to anti-epileptic drugs.

Anti-epileptic drug treatment following a first seizure

The first time that a person is offered anti-epileptic drug treatment might be after their first seizure. A number of trials have been undertaken that compare starting or not starting anti-epileptic drug treatment following a first seizure. These trials have shown that starting an anti-epileptic drug reduces the chance of a second seizure. For example, on average after two years, the risk of a second seizure is around 30 per cent with anti-epileptic drug treatment and around 40 per cent without, thus the effect of treatment is relatively small—around 10 per cent difference. There are some patients for whom the risk of recurrence is higher, such as those with an abnormal EEG and/or brain scan, but the benefit of treatment is also higher for these individuals. Whilst anti-epileptic drugs might reduce the risk of a seizure recurrence, they are also associated with a number of side-effects as discussed below. For people who have had a first seizure there is a trade-off between the relatively small benefit of starting treatment and the possibility of side-effects. It is important that patient and doctor have a discussion about these trade-offs to help the patient or the family of a young child, make a decision as to whether they would want to start treatment or not.

Anti-epileptic drug treatment following a diagnosis of epilepsy

Once a person has had two or more seizures and given a diagnosis of epilepsy, they will usually be advised to start treatment with an anti-epileptic drug. However, some may choose not to start treatment, particularly if their seizures have been brief and caused minor symptoms (for example, simple partial seizures). Here again, the doctor and patient and/or carers must have a discussion about the potential benefits and trade-offs of the treatment thought most appropriate for the patient according to their seizure type and epilepsy syndrome. In terms of benefit, on average, seizures will eventually stop for 60–70 per cent of patients starting anti-epileptic drug treatment, whilst the main trade-offs are the possible side-effects, which are discussed below. Because of the relatively small but important risk of causing abnormalities in the developing foetus (see below), particular attention must be paid to women of child-bearing age.

Which anti-epileptic drug should be used?

There are numerous anti-epileptic drugs available as outlined in Table 6.1. Some are thought to be more effective than others for certain seizure types and epilepsy syndromes, and there is increasing evidence from clinical trials to support this. One of the first things to consider, therefore, when choosing a treatment is how effective it is likely to be at controlling seizures. A second factor to consider is the side-effects that might occur. The drugs do differ in some of the side-effects that might occur and people will differ in the sort of side-effects that might be acceptable. For example, a drug that might cause weight gain might be unacceptable to someone who is overweight, but acceptable to someone that is underweight. Similarly some drugs are thought more likely to cause abnormalities in the developing child (foetus) than others. A third factor to consider is how easy the drug is to administer, for example, does it need to be taken multiple times per day or can it be taken in a form other than tablet, for example, liquid, or sprinkle formulation that can be sprinkled over food. This can be particularly important for children, who may not like taking medicine or are unable to swallow tablets and capsules.

Each drug has two names—the generic or chemical name (for example, sodium valproate), and the brand name (for example, Epilim), which is the name given by the maker of the drug. When a drug first becomes available it is manufactured by only one drug company under patent. Once the patent runs out, usually after a few years, other companies are allowed to make that drug as well. These companies usually sell the drug at a much cheaper price, and they may sell the drug by its generic name or use another brand name. For example, at the time or writing, there are a number of companies manufacturing lamotrigine (generic name), which on the packaging may be called lamotrigine and/or one of numerous brand names. Doctors may write a prescription using either the generic or trade name. If the generic name is used, the pharmacist in the retail chemist or hospital pharmacy department can provide either the generic or brand drug. If, however, the doctor prescribes the drug using the brand name, then the pharmacist must provide the patient with that brand.

Table 6.1 shows the anti-epileptic drugs which are currently available, using generic and trade names, the various preparations of the drug, and the usual adult daily dosage. It is difficult to provide a guide for children's dosages, as the right dose must be based on the age of the child and their weight. When children reach 12 or 13 years of age, the anti-epileptic drugs are then usually prescribed in an adult dose, although usually at the lower end of the adult dose range. The drugs most commonly used as first line treatment are denoted with *.

Table 6.1 Anti-epileptic drugs

Generic name	Brand name	Preparations	Adult doses
Acetazolamide	Diamox	250mg tablets 250mg capsules	250mg to 1000mg per day taken in two divided doses
*Carbamazepine	Tegretol	100mg, 200mg, 400mg tablets 100mg, 200mg chew tablets 200mg, 400mg Retard tablets (slow release) 100mg/5 ml sugar-free syrup	400mg to 1000mg per day taken in two divided doses
Clobazam	Frisium	10mg tablets (some hospital pharmacies can make smaller tablets or liquid preparations)	10mg to 40mg per day taken in two divided doses
Clonazepam	Rivotril, Clonopil	0.5mg, 2.0mg tablets	0.5mg to 4mg per day taken in two or three divided doses
Ethosuximide	Zarontin, Emeside	250mg capsules, 250mg/5ml syrup (Zarontin only available as liquid)	500mg to 2000mg per day taken in two or three divided doses
Gabapentin	Neurontin	100mg, 300mg, 400mg, 600mg capsules.	900mg to 3600mg per day taken in two or three divided doses
*Lamotrigine	Lamictal	25mg, 50mg, 100mg, 200mg tablets. 2mg, 5mg, 25mg, 100mg dispersible tablets	Patients not taking valproate: 100mg to 500mg per day taken in two divided doses Patients taking valproate: 100mg to 200mg per day taken in two divided doses
Levetiracetam	Keppra	250mg, 500mg, 750mg, 100mg tablets 100mg/ml solution	500mg to 3000mg per day taken in two divided doses
Oxcarbazepine	Trileptal	150mg, 300mg, 600mg tablets 300mg/5ml suspension	600mg to 2000mg per day taken in two divided doses

(continued)

Table 6.1 Anti-epileptic drugs *(continued)*

Generic name	Brand name	Preparations	Adult doses
Phenobarbital	Gardenal, Luminal	15mg, 30mg, 60mg, 100mg tabs. 30mg/10 ml syrup	60mg to 200mg per day taken in two divided doses
*Phenytoin	Epanutin, Dilantin	25mg, 50mg, 100mg, 300mg tablets 25mg chewable tablets	200mg to 300mg per day taken in two divided doses
Pregabalin	Lyrica	25mg, 50mg, 75mg, 100mg, 200mg, 300mg tablets	150mg to 600mg per day taken in two divided doses
Primidone	Mysoline	250mg tablets	500mg to 1500mg per day taken in two divided doses
Rufinamide	Inovelon	100mg, 200mg, 400mg tablets	1000mg to 1800mg per day taken in two divided doses
Tiagabine	Gabitril	5mg, 10mg, 15mg tablets	15mg to 45mg per day taken in three divided doses
Topiramate	Topamax	25mg, 50mg, 100mg, 200mg tablets	100mg to 400mg per day taken in two divided doses.
*Valproate	Epilim, Orlept, Episenta, Epilim chronospheres, Convulex, Depakine, Depakote, Depomide	100mg, 200mg, 500mg tablets 50mg, 100mg, 250mg, 500mg 750mg, chronosphere capsules 200mg, 300mg, 500mg Chrono tablets (slow release) 150mg, 300mg, 500mg capsules	600mg to 2000mg per day taken in two divided doses
Vigabatrin	Sabril	500mg tablets; a sachet containing powder and 500mg per sachet	1000mg to 2500mg per day taken in two divided doses
Zonisamide	Zonegran	25mg, 50mg, 100mg tablets	100mg to 500mg per day taken in two divided doses

Table 6.2 shows the generic name of the drug, the types of epilepsy or seizures which each drug is used to treat, and the side-effects that may be associated with the drugs. The drugs most commonly used as first line treatments are denoted by*.

Table 6.2

Generic name	Seizure types	Side-effects****
Acetazolamide	Add-on for focal** seizures and for seizures that cluster around menstrual periods	Nausea, vomiting, pins and needles/tingling when used in high doses
*Carbamazepine	Drug of choice for focal** seizures	Nausea and vomiting, dizziness, drowsiness, headache, unsteadiness, confusion, blurred or double vision, rash, low white blood cell count.
Clobazam	Add-on for focal** or generalized*** seizures. Also used when seizures cluster around menstrual periods	Drowsiness, confusion, unsteadiness
Clonazepam	Add-on for focal** or generalized*** seizures	Drowsiness, confusion, unsteadiness
Ethosuximide	Monotherapy or add-on for absence seizures; may also be effective for myoclonic seizures	Nausea, vomiting, headache, diarrhoea, abdominal pain, reduced appetite
Gabapentin	Add-on for focal** seizures	Drowsiness, lethargy, nausea, weight gain
*Lamotrigine	Drug of choice for focal** seizures Also used for generalized*** seizures especially in women when attempting to avoid valproate	Rash and other allergic reactions, liver dysfunction, nausea, vomiting, headache, fatigue, dizziness, sleep disturbances, tremor, agitation, confusion,
Levetiracetam	Focal** or generalized*** seizures	Nausea, vomiting, indigestion weight changes, drowsiness, unsteadiness and dizziness, emotional lability, insomnia, anxiety, aggression and irritability

(continued)

Table 6.2 (*continued*)

Generic name	Seizure types	Side-effects****
Oxcarbazepine	Focal** seizures	Nausea, vomiting, constipation, diarrhoea, abdominal pain, dizziness, headache, drowsiness, agitation, unsteadiness, confusion, impaired concentration, rash, double or blurred vision
Phenobarbital	Focal** or generalized*** seizures	Liver dysfunction, jaundice, behavioural disturbances, irritability, drowsiness, lethargy, depression, unsteadiness, impaired memory, rash
*Phenytoin	Focal** seizures	Nausea, vomiting, constipation, insomnia, dizziness, headache, gum swelling, rash, acne, facial hair, coarsening of facial features
Pregabalin	Add-on for focal** seizures	Dry mouth, constipation, nausea, vomiting, dizziness, drowsiness, irritability, reduced memory and concentration, fatigue, weight gain
Primidone	Focal*** or generalized*** seizures	Liver dysfunction, jaundice, behavioural disturbances, irritability, drowsiness, lethargy, depression, unsteadiness, impaired memory, rash
Rufinamide	Atonic (drop) and tonic (stiffening) seizures, particularly in Lennox–Gastaut syndrome	Drowsiness, dizziness, headache
Tiagabine	Add-on for focal** seizures	Diarrhoea, dizziness, tiredness, nervousness, tremor, impaired concentration, emotional lability, speech impairment
Topiramate	Focal** or generalized*** seizures	Nausea, abdominal pain, weight loss, headache, fatigue, dizziness, speech difficulty, reduced concentration and memory, anxiety, depression
*Valproate	First-line treatment for generalized*** seizures. Also used for focal seizure	Gastric irritation, diarrhoea, weight gain, hyperammonaemia, thrombocytopenia, transient hair loss

(*continued*)

Table 6.2 (*continued*)

Generic name	Seizure types	Side-effects****
Vigabatrin	First line treatment for infantile spasms (West syndrome)*; drug of last choice in focal seizures	Increased appetite, irritability, visual field constriction (possibly irreversible)
Zonisamide	Add-on for focal** or generalized*** seizures	Nausea, diarrhoea, abdominal pain, reduced appetite, weight loss, drowsiness, dizziness, confusion, agitation, irritability, depression, unsteadiness, impaired memory and attention, double vision and rash

* First-line treatments
**Focal seizures include simple partial, complex partial and secondary generalized tonic–clonic seizures
***Generalized seizures include generalized tonic–clonic seizure, myoclonic seizures and absence seizures
****The list of side-effects is not exhaustive, but gives a range of side-effects that might be seen.
  Although the list might be frightening at first glance, many patients have little in the way of
  side-effects, and most of the side-effects are dose-related, in other words they occur when higher doses
  are used.

Tables 6.1 and 6.2 describe all the common anti-epileptic drugs which may be given by mouth. There are a number of other drugs which are used only in status epilepticus (Chapter 2), when they are then given by either an injection into a vein (intravenous route) or by administering a special solution into the rectum or buccal cavity. These drugs include chlormethiazole (Heminevrin), lignocaine (Xylocard), paraldehyde (no trade name). Diazepam (Valium) and lorazepam (Ativan) are probably the most frequently employed drugs in the UK. Another drug, midazolam (called Hypnovel or Epistatus), is being increasingly used for patients that have clusters of seizures or prolonged seizures. When this occurs, it can be injected into the mouth by carers into the space between the teeth and cheek (called the buccal cavity) where it is quickly absorbed. If diazepam or midazolam are given either rectally or buccally, then they can prevent repeated admissions to hospital.

The side-effects of the anti-epileptic drugs

The main side-effects of all the anti-epileptic drugs are summarized in Table 6.2. Generally, there are potentially three types of side-effects which may be associated with any drug, including anti-epileptic drugs.

Allergic or hypersensitive (idiosyncratic) side-effects

These are rare and occur usually within one or two weeks of starting the drug. The effects are usually unpredictable, and, once they have occurred, it means that the drug must be stopped and can probably not be used again. The most common side-effect of this type is a widespread, itchy rash. This occurs in about 5 per cent of patients soon after starting on an anti-epileptic drug. The drugs which tend to cause rashes are carbamazepine, lamotrigine, phenobarbital, and phenytoin.

Dose-related side-effects

These may be caused by either introducing the drug too quickly or by giving too much. Most of the anti-epileptic drugs can cause such side-effects, which include drowsiness, unsteadiness, nausea, blurred or double vision. These effects can be avoided by starting the drug more slowly; they disappear if the dose is reduced. Doctors will usually start a patient on a low dose and build up the dose over a few weeks to what is called a maintenance dose, usually at the low end of the dose range. If seizures recur, then the dose is increased in stages until either the seizures are controlled or side-effects occur. If the person continues to have seizures and has side-effects then options include switching to another treatment or reducing the dose and adding a second treatment.

On average, epilepsy in the elderly is more likely to be controlled with drugs than it is for younger adults; approximately 70-75% of people over the age of 65 years will have their epilepsy controlled. However, the overall prognosis and quality of life for the individual will depend very much upon the cause of the epilepsy. Treating seizures will not affect the growth of a brain tumour, nor will it stop the advance of Alzheimer's disease or reduce the disability caused by a stroke.

An elderly person presenting with epilepsy is likely to be taking medicine for other medical conditions. When choosing an antiepileptic drug it is important to take this into account as there may be important interactions between drugs, meaning that some antiepileptic drugs should probably be avoided. The elderly are often more likely to experience side-effects of antiepileptic drug treatment and they will usually require a lower starting dose than would be given to younger adults. Finally, it is best to try and avoid using antiepileptic medications that may cause neurological side-effects that might affect their balance, movement, memory and mood. Specific antiepileptic medications that should either be avoided or used with great caution in the elderly include phenytoin, carbamazepine and topiramate.

Long term or chronic side-effects

These are side-effects that develop more slowly, over months or years. They are more common in patients taking more than one drug, and often in high doses. Once again, the effects may be more difficult to recognize (by both the patient and doctor), as they tend to develop gradually and do not cause any acute or sudden problem. The older drugs such as phenobarbital, primidone, and phenytoin, and one of the newer drugs, vigabatrin, are probably more likely to cause chronic, or long-term, side-effects, whilst the newer anti-epileptic drugs are thought to be safer, although many of the newer drugs have not been available long enough for their longer-term side-effects to be thoroughly assessed.

One of the most common concerns of patients and parents of children who are receiving anti-epileptic drugs is the effect of drugs on school or work performance, memory, mood, and behaviour. Anti-epileptic drugs may cause some initial drowsiness or changes in mood and behaviour, as the drug is being started, but these effects usually wear off. The older anti-epileptic drugs such as phenobarbital and phenytoin have been shown to reduce a patient's concentration or attention span and therefore cause problems in memory, particularly short-term memory. This, in turn can adversely affect learning and the ability to do certain tasks. These problems are thought less likely to occur with drugs such as carbamazepine and sodium valproate as well as many of the newer drugs. It is often difficult to determine whether a problem with either learning or behaviour is definitely due to a drug. A number of patients, in addition to having epilepsy, may also have learning and behavioural difficulties as other manifestations of the brain problems that are causing epilepsy. Also, frequent seizures can affect memory as well as behaviour.

Due to their side-effects, phenytoin and phenobarbital are now rarely used as first-line treatments, particularly in developed countries that can afford alternatives. However, phenytoin remains a commonly used drug in the USA. Phenytoin has an unfortunate effect on the gums, which tend to thicken and grow down between the teeth. This can sometimes be reduced by twice daily brushing upwards and downwards with a medium bristle tooth brush. If necessary, a dentist can push back the gums or remove the excessive tissue. This overgrowth of gum tissue is reflected in subtle changes in the lips and facial skin, which may become slightly 'fleshy'. Phenytoin and barbiturates predispose the person to acne of the face and back, and may cause some slight excess of facial hair. These cosmetic effects may be a reason to avoid using these drugs in young people. Phenobarbital might affect the shoulder joint in a few people, so that it becomes stiff and painful. In others, changes in the tendons of the hands and connective tissue of the palms leads to a contracture (Dupuytren's contracture) of the hands. Phenytoin and even some of the other anti-epileptic drugs used over a number of years may cause an excessive metabolism of the body's vitamin D supplies, which may lead to osteoporosis and rickets, in the absence of adequate diet or sunlight (which helps form vitamin D).

Finally, and importantly, there is the issue of the effect of anti-epileptic drugs on the developing baby—a particular concern to women with epilepsy. Since anti-epileptic drug treatment lasts for many years, it is important that this issue is discussed with young women when they start anti-epileptic drug treatment, even if they are not considering pregnancy at that time. It is important to stress that the great majority of pregnancies for women with epilepsy go without complication. However, there is a slight increase in the occurrence of foetal abnormalities for babies born to mothers with epilepsy and taking anti-epileptic drugs. From the analysis of a large number of patients, it is clear that much of this increase is due to anti-epileptic drugs, and the average risk of a major malformation is around 5 per cent (in other words one in twenty) for women taking one anti-epileptic drug. This risk might go up to 10 per cent (one in ten) for women taking two drugs. Malformations might include a cleft-(hare) lip or palate, heart defects and spina bifida. Most of these malformations can be picked up on ultrasound scans during pregnancy. Some malformations are more common with certain drugs, for example, spina bifida is more common with valproate. Studies have suggested that the risk of a major malformation is higher with valproate than with the other commonly used drugs. More recently valproate has also been associated with speech and learning difficulties in children where the mothers have taken it during pregnancy. The learning difficulties seem to particularly affect speech and language and may occur without the child having any major malformations. This can make it difficult for young women with generalized epilepsy to choose their first treatment, as valproate has been shown to be the best drug to control seizures, whilst it is probably the most harmful first-line drug in pregnancy. It is also important to realize that if a mother has frequent generalized tonic–clonic seizures during pregnancy this may actually cause harm to mother and/or baby. For the majority of women with epilepsy who are planning a pregnancy, the advice will be to take anti-epileptic drug treatment, aiming for the lowest dose that can control seizures, and treatment with one drug, if possible. These issues should all be discussed with women when treatment is started, before they are planning any pregnancy, and where possible, women should be encouraged to plan the pregnancy. All women with epilepsy who are considering having children, should be taking folic acid (one of the B vitamins), as it is thought that this can reduce the risk of spina bifida.

How is the anti-epileptic drug to be given?

The most appropriate drug for the patient's seizure type or epilepsy syndrome must be given in the preparation which is most acceptable to the patient. For adult patients, this will usually be in tablet or capsule form, for young children it will be a flavoured liquid or syrup (preferably sugar-free in order to avoid tooth decay) or a tablet or powder that dissolves completely in water or juice. Most drugs (in whichever preparation) need to be given twice, or rarely, three times a day in order to maintain as steady a state as possible in the blood. Because phenobarbital and phenytoin are so slowly broken down in the body, these drugs can be given only once a day. When given two or three times a day, each dose should be more or less the same in order to avoid any dose-related side-effects, which are more likely if one large dose is given. Dose-related side-effects may be avoided by the use of sustained or controlled-release preparations. Sustained or controlled-release means that the drug is released more slowly into the blood from the bowel. This reduces the chance of acute dose-related side-effects such as unsteadiness, vomiting, sedation, double vision, or tremor. Examples of such preparations are Tegretol Retard, Episenta and Epilim Chrono.

As far as possible, only one anti-epileptic drug should be prescribed at a time (monotherapy). Most patients, both children and adults, will have their epilepsy controlled by a single drug. The remainder, perhaps 30 per cent of these patients, will need to take two or even (very rarely), three anti-epileptic drugs (polytherapy). The choice of a second drug again depends upon the type of seizure and known side-effects of the drugs, and any interaction between the two. As an example, in childhood absence epilepsy (previously called petit mal), the first choice drug would be sodium valproate. If seizures were not fully controlled on this drug, the first step would be to consider whether the dose was adequate. Only then would a second choice drug be added, probably ethosuximide or lamotrigine.

Drug interactions—which other drugs can be safely taken with anti-epileptic drugs?

Patients with epilepsy experience other illnesses or infections like anyone else, and have to take additional drugs to treat them. This includes taking antibiotics for infections, analgesics for pain relief (for example, headaches), or treatment for asthma. Many women will also want to use the contraceptive pill. Most drugs can be taken safely with all the anti-epileptic drugs; however, there are one or two important exceptions, some of which are outlined below:

◆ carbamazepine, phenytoin, phenobarbital, topiramate, and rufinamide interfere with the effectiveness of the oral contraceptive pill, leading to less reliable contraception. Women taking the combined oral contraceptive pill will need to take a higher dose and should seek advice from their doctor or family planning service.

◆ lamotrigine is affected by the combined oral contraceptive pill, which reduces the amount of lamotrigine in the blood. It is particularly important for women taking lamotrigine who subsequently start taking it with a contraceptive pill.

◆ sodium valproate and aspirin may interact and cause excessive bleeding after a cut or minor injury.

◆ theophylline (used in asthma) may reduce the effectiveness of carbamazepine, leading to increased seizures.

◆ certain antibiotics can reduce the effectiveness of some anti-epileptic drugs.

It is important that people with epilepsy tell their doctor about any other drugs that they are taking. Interactions between the drugs may provide an explanation for some side-effects or for an increase in seizure frequency or status epilepticus (Chapter 2).

When patients are taking more than one anti-epileptic drug, this increases the risk of developing side-effects, particularly if phenytoin is one of the drugs. Any changes in the doses of the two drugs must be made gradually and the patient may rarely need to have blood levels of the drugs measured at intervals.

When should another anti-epileptic drug be given?

As mentioned above, the first choice drug should be used alone (monotherapy) and in the lowest dose to control seizures without producing any unacceptable side-effects. If the initial control of seizures is less than complete, then the dose of that drug should be increased gradually until either complete control is achieved, or side-effects develop. If unacceptable side-effects occur before control is reached, then there are two alternatives:

◆ if seizure control has been poor a different drug can be used to replace the first drug, or an additional drug can be added to the first drug. Which alternative is chosen depends on the individual patient and also on the doctor.

◆ if there has been some reasonable control with the first drug, it might be appropriate to add a second anti-epileptic drug without withdrawing the first drug. If complete seizure control is then achieved, the patient will have the option of trying to withdraw the first drug, although this would be at the risk of seizures recurring. If the initial drug has been ineffective, it would be appropriate to simultaneously replace the first drug with the second.

Treatment with three or more anti-epileptic drugs is rarely beneficial and is often associated with significant side-effects.

How is treatment monitored—including blood levels of drugs?

Any patient's response to treatment with anti-epileptic drugs is based, first, on whether the seizures have reduced in frequency or stopped completely, and secondly, whether there have been any side-effects. If a patient has good seizure control but unacceptable side-effects then the dose of the drug should be reduced slightly in the expectation that seizure control will continue, but the adverse effects become less prominent. If the patient has some, but not complete seizure control and no side-effects, then the dose is increased. Therefore, a patient is receiving the correct dose of the drug when the seizures have stopped and there are no side-effects. In the past, doctors used to emphasize the importance of blood tests to measure the amount of drug in the blood (called therapeutic blood level monitoring). This is because there is some relationship between the blood level of the drug and its therapeutic and toxic effects. That is to say, there are blood levels of anti-epileptic drugs below which therapeutic effects do not occur (the drug is unlikely to be effective), and above which no further benefit is achieved without causing toxicity. However, the lowest and highest levels in the blood are only approximate guidelines, and for the majority of patients, the measurement of blood levels of anti-epileptic drugs is not necessary, indeed inappropriate measurement can result in harm. For example, a patient may have little in the way of side-effects and have their seizures controlled on a dose of treatment that is associated with blood levels above the therapeutic range; an unwary or inexperienced doctor might check the blood levels for this patient and then advise a reduction in dose. This could result in recurrence of seizures, which can be devastating, particularly for someone that has regained their driving licence having gone a year or more without seizures.

There are many factors which affect the blood levels of anti-epileptic drugs, including the chemical structure of the drug and how it is carried in the blood (usually attached to proteins); the age and sex of the patient; an individual's metabolism of the drug (by either the kidney or liver, and whether there is any disease of these organs); and how regularly and reliably the drug is taken. Because of all these factors, the lack of a clear correlation between blood levels and effectiveness or toxicity, and the fact that a blood test may be distressing (particularly for children), doctors are now less inclined to monitor anti-epileptic drug blood levels. However, there are certain situations where measuring blood levels may be important, including:

- where there is the possibility of the patient not taking the drug as prescribed. This is one of the most common reasons for poor seizure control. Measuring the blood level of the drug will go some way to confirm or exclude this possibility. The reason for wanting to check the blood level must be discussed with the patient.

- if the patient presents in status epilepticus, that is, in a prolonged seizure

- if the patient has severe learning difficulties and is not able to tell the doctor of side-effects

- if the patient is taking phenytoin, particularly with another anti-epileptic drug. This is because the metabolism of phenytoin is different from all other anti-epileptic drugs. A small change in dosage, either up or down respectively, may result in toxicity and side-effects or loss of control of seizures

- special situations, including pregnancy, or when there is a disorder of the kidney or liver. This is because these three situations may significantly affect how the drug is metabolized in the body.

How to help children and adults take their drugs regularly

If a drug is to be taken reliably and regularly, a patient must be fully informed about that drug, including the likely benefit, side-effects, and possible consequences of not taking it regularly. A plan of the proposed management and possible side-effects of the anti-epileptic drug must be discussed with the patient (or family) at diagnosis and at the outset of treatment. Ideally the patient should be given both oral and written information about their treatment and treatment plan. It is unreasonable to expect patients to remember all that has been discussed during a consultation, especially when upset or anxious. Written information can reinforce what has been discussed and help prevent misunderstandings.

What else may be used to treat epilepsy?

The use of anti-epileptic drugs is clearly the principal method of treating epilepsy. In those situations where a specific cause for the seizures has been found, then other treatments may be necessary and below we discuss surgical approaches to treating epilepsy. There are also other non-drug treatments,

113

such as dietary manipulation, which may help people whose epilepsy proves difficult to control with drugs.

Dietary manipulation

There have been a number of attempts to control epileptic seizures by modifying the diet. This arose from the observation many years ago that fasting or starvation seemed to be associated with a reduction in the frequency of seizures. In the fasting state, normal metabolism is altered with the appearance of substances in the blood and urine, called ketones, which are created when the body metabolizes fat. It is not known how or why ketones are linked with seizure control. Of course, there may be no direct relationship between the two, and the occurrence of the two together may be coincidental. There is a diet which produces ketones, but without the patient having to be starved. The diet has some similarities to the Atkins diet and is very rich in fat and oils, which makes it rather unpalatable. Because 70 per cent of the diet is in this fat form (the remaining 30 per cent coming from protein and carbohydrate), extra vitamins and minerals (such as calcium and magnesium) must be given. In spite of all the fat and oil eaten in this diet, there is no change in the blood level of cholesterol which is responsible for causing coronary heart disease. The main disadvantages with this diet are its rather unpleasant taste and texture; it causes diarrhoea or constipation, and the fact that the diet must be strictly followed. Its use is usually restricted to infants and children with very severe epilepsy with multiple and usually generalized seizures (often with the Lennox–Gastaut and severe myoclonic epilepsy syndromes). Although a recent trial has proved that this diet is effective in the short term, we still do not know whether it is effective at controlling seizures in the long term, nor whether there are any longer-term health problems caused by the diet. One of the major benefits of the ketogenic diet is that, if it is effective, then one or more of the child's anti-epileptic drugs can be gradually stopped with a reduction in side-effects. However, most children whose seizures are well controlled on the diet will still need to keep taking at least one anti-epileptic drug.

There are few, extremely rare conditions, where the epilepsy is caused by an inborn error of metabolism. This means that either the body is missing, or is unable to use, a particular substance, usually a vitamin or enzyme, and, as a result the person develops epilepsy, and often other problems (for example, skin rashes, loss of hair, failure to grow). If the missing substance is then given in large doses, then the epilepsy may stop. Examples of these conditions include pyridoxine (vitamin B6)-dependent seizures, and biotinidase deficiency, both of which usually begin by affecting babies or infants in the first few days or weeks of life.

Surgery

The surgical treatment of epilepsy is becoming increasingly useful, particularly when the seizures are not controlled by anti-epileptic drugs. However, surgery must only be undertaken after a careful detailed assessment of the patient. This, and the operation, should only be carried out in recognized specialist centres. This is because both the assessment of the patient and the operation itself involve expert and sophisticated procedures—and clearly surgery is an irreversible treatment.

Surgical treatment depends on two main principles or ideas:

- the first is that a local abnormal area of brain can be entirely removed, leaving behind only healthy, normal brain (this is called resection).

- the second is that the spread of the seizure discharge (to involve other parts of the brain as is illustrated in Figure 2.1), can be prevented by cutting the nerve fibre which cause the discharge (this is called disconnection or transection).

Penfield and Rasmussen, two Canadian neurosurgeons, were the pioneers of surgery for epilepsy and much of the surgical assessment and treatment of patients today is based on their early work. One of the most important questions that must be answered before surgery can be considered is: from where precisely within the brain do the seizures originate? When the cause is a tumour or cyst, then this is relatively easy to answer, but frequently the cause is an area of brain that developed abnormally in foetal life. The identification of the abnormal part of the brain relies upon magnetic resonance imaging, and the use of special electrodes to try and record or 'capture' the epileptic discharge. The scalp electrodes (used in a routine EEG) are not usually sensitive enough for this task, and so other electrodes, called depth electrodes (which are inserted into the brain) may be used, or a cluster of electrodes (a grid or mat) might be placed over the surface of the brain. Because these special electrodes are in very close contact with the brain, there is a much greater chance that they will pick up the epileptic discharge. In addition to these assessments, people being considered for surgery usually also need detailed psychological evaluation, specifically to try and identify which side of the brain is responsible for language and memory, so that these areas are not damaged during the operation. Consideration must also be given to avoid operating in those parts of the brain responsible for movement; it would be unacceptable to stop the seizures at the expense of causing a paralysis on one side of the body (hemiplegia), which might result in losing the ability to walk or write, or loss of speech.

Before a patient is considered for surgical treatment of their epilepsy, it must be shown that the patient's seizures cannot be adequately controlled using anti-epileptic drugs. It is unwise to operate too early, as the epilepsy might remit (stop) spontaneously, although this is unlikely in the difficult epilepsies. However, if surgery is delayed for too long, then this may limit the potential success of the operation because the patient has suffered irreversible educational and social consequences of repeated seizures. Most specialists would now consider that if acceptable seizure control has not been achieved using optimal doses of anti-epileptic drugs after one, or no more than two years, then surgery should be considered as the next step in a patient's treatment. It has been estimated that many patients in the UK might currently benefit from surgery. There are four types of surgical procedure that are currently undertaken:

◆ removing a large, identifiable lesion such as an area of abnormal brain development, tumour or cyst.

◆ removing an entire cerebral hemisphere. This is done when the whole of one side of the brain is abnormal, this being associated with hemiplegia (weakness down one side of the body). The operation sounds dramatic, but is often successful leading to a complete resolution of seizures and, frequently, an improvement in the hemiplegia. Hemispherectomy is particularly useful in children with the Sturge–Weber syndrome (Chapter 3) and in Rasmussen syndrome (Chapter 2).

◆ removing a small or large lesion which has been identified on the basis of detailed specialized EEG recording and imaging. This procedure is the one frequently used in temporal lobe epilepsy, where different parts and amounts of the temporal lobe are removed. Advances in imaging have led to the identification of subtle structural abnormalities in not just the temporal lobes, but also the frontal lobes which are responsible for seizures.

◆ carrying out a disconnection procedure; this is to try and separate the focus (site of abnormal electrical activity) of origin of the seizure from other parts of the brain, by cutting the nerve fibres which allow the epileptic discharge to spread. Operations attempted have included division (cutting) of the corpus callosum. This is a large band of fibre which transmits electrical information from one hemisphere to another. A more sophisticated, technically difficult procedure (called subpial transection) appears to be more successful.

◆ vagal nerve stimulation. This does not involve brain surgery. In some way this procedure is like having a pacemaker fitted. A battery (the size of a large wrist watch) is implanted under the skin on the left side of the chest, and connected to a wire the other end of which is connected to the vagus nerve in the neck. This treatment is palliative, in that it reduces the frequency of seizures for around a third of patients, but would not be expected to stop seizures completely. Unfortunately, the positive effects of vagal nerve stimulation may not be seen for up to six or even twelve months after it has been implanted.

Overall, the results of epilepsy surgery are encouraging, as many as 60–70 per cent of people who have operations for epilepsy have no further seizures, whilst another 10–20 per cent are much improved. Patients undergoing a hemispherectomy or temporal lobectomy do better than patients who have an operation on their frontal lobe or a corpus callosotomy. For some patients who have had to live with uncontrolled seizures for many years, a cure of their epilepsy following surgery may come as something of a shock, requiring a major adjustment in their lives. These patients need careful and expert support and counselling. For many, but not all, patients whose seizures stop after one of the surgical procedures described above, anti-epileptic drugs may also eventually be discontinued.

Other treatments

These include hypnosis, aromatherapy, bio-feedback, homeopathy, and acupuncture. The success of these techniques, for which there is little or no scientific evidence of effectiveness, is variable and limited. However, patients may find them of value in giving a sense of control over their bodies and their lives.

General principles

The treatment of epilepsy extends far beyond the prescription of anti-epileptic medication. It is, of course, important to correctly identify the type of epilepsy and to prescribe the most appropriate anti-epileptic drug to obtain the best possible control of seizures without side-effects. However, for many patients and their families, social and psychological factors far outweigh the problem of preventing or controlling the seizures. Help may best be given through a multidisciplinary approach, preferably within a specialist clinic with advice from a number of different specialists, including nurses, psychologists, and psychiatrists. Many patients get practical help and support from voluntary associations including Epilepsy Action (previously, British Epilepsy Association), the National Society for Epilepsy and Epilepsy Bereaved, and patients should be informed of their address and telephone number. A list of these and other associations and their addresses appears in Appendix 2.

Treatment of special situations

Status epilepticus

Occasionally, a single, generalized tonic–clonic or generalized absence (petit mal) seizure may be prolonged (lasting more than 30 minutes) or the seizures may follow each other in rapid succession without full recovery between each one. When this happens, it is called status epilepticus (also see Chapter 2). There are a number of different types of status epilepticus, the most common being:

Type of status epilepticus	Seizure characteristics
Convulsive status	Prolonged tonic–clonic seizure
Non-convulsive status (non-convulsive means that there are no jerks or abnormal movements; it can also be called electrical status epilepticus)	a) prolonged absence seizure b) prolonged complex partial seizure
Epilepsia partialis continua (this is rare)	Continuous twitching of one arm/leg or one side of the face, or both (this may last for minutes, hours, days or weeks)

The EEG is not usually required in convulsive status, as the diagnosis is obvious. The EEG may be extremely valuable in helping to diagnose non-convulsive or electrical status. In this type of status, the diagnosis of epilepsy may not be immediately obvious. The patients may just appear confused or bewildered, with some inappropriate behaviour. An EEG recorded at this time will confirm the diagnosis. Non-convulsive status occurs more commonly in children and young people with the more serious epilepsy syndromes, including Lennox–Gastaut syndrome and myoclonic–astatic epilepsy and also in epilepsy caused by some genetic factors such as Rett and Angelman syndromes. Non-convulsive status epilepticus may be particularly difficult to recognize in these people because they usually have significant learning difficulties and behaviour problems. This is why the EEG may be very important in making the correct diagnosis.

Convulsive status epilepticus is a medical emergency that requires prompt treatment. When a convulsion is prolonged, or a patient does not recover fully between seizures, there is a danger that a lack of an adequate oxygen supply to the brain may cause brain damage. There is also the risk of vomiting with aspiration of the vomit into the lungs which can also reduce the supply of oxygen to the brain. Although rare, patients may die in status epilepticus. The longer the patient has been in status epilepticus, the harder it is to stop it. Treatment consists of giving a fast-acting anti-epileptic drug as quickly as possible. This is usually given into a vein, or if this is difficult (which may be the case in young children), into the rectum or buccal cavity. The most commonly used drugs are diazepam (also called Valium, Diazemuls, or in a rectal tube preparation, Stesolid) and lorazapam (Ativan). Rectal diazepam may be given by parents or carers at home, but increasingly another drug, midazolam, is being used. Midazolam (Hypnovel or Epistatus) can be injected into the mouth in the space between the teeth and gums (buccal cavity). Midazolam is therefore easier to administer and more socially acceptable than giving rectal diazepam. Both rectal diazepam and buccal midazolam are useful treatments as they can be given by parents or carers at home or in a school or college. Other drugs that are sometimes used in hospital include chlormethiazole (Heminevrin), and paraldehyde. Paraldehyde is usually given via the rectum but may, very rarely, be administered as an intramuscular injection into the buttocks. Paraldehyde is a very effective anti-epileptic drug but its main disadvantage is its unpleasant smell.

If the first dose of diazepam, midazolam, lorazepam, or paraldehyde does not terminate the status, then a second dose may be given. If this is not successful, then the patient must be treated more urgently, and admitted to the intensive care unit. This is because the suppression of the seizure may require such considerable amounts of drugs that normal breathing may also be suppressed. In this situation, patients may require ventilator-assisted respiration, and intensive nursing. The longer-acting drugs which are most commonly used include phenytoin and phenobarbital. They are usually given by a drip intravenously to ensure that they work quickly. As the seizure comes under control, drugs can be given again by mouth.

Once the patient has recovered and is stable, any factors which may have caused the status epilepticus must be identified to try and prevent a recurrence. In many situations, this will involve a review of the person's usual oral anti-epileptic medication, and ensuring that patients take their medication regularly.

Infantile spasms

Infantile spasms are a rare type of epileptic seizure that usually affects infants between 3 and 9 months of age. This type of epilepsy, or epilepsy syndrome, is called West syndrome (Chapter 2). There are at least fifty causes of West syndrome and the outcome of children with this epilepsy syndrome depends almost as much as the underlying cause as the success of its treatment. The treatment of infantile spasms is unlike that of other epilepsies. Treatment usually consists of giving an anti-epileptic drug called vigabatrin, or a steroid. Vigabatrin is usually given as a powder which dissolves completely in water, milk or juice. Vigabatrin is usually given twice a day and for about 4 or 6 months. The steroid can either be given by an intramuscular injection or by mouth. The drug which is given by injection is called ACTH (adrenocorticotrophic hormone) or tetracosactide, and by mouth, prednisolone. Both tetracosactide (the intramuscular injection) and prednisolone (the tablet) are usually given once (rarely twice) a day for at least two to three weeks until the spasms have stopped, and then every other day, and eventually just once a week. Only about one half to two-thirds of children will respond to either vigabatrin or to ACTH or prednisolone. Children who have infantile spasms that are caused by the condition tuberous sclerosis respond very well to treatment with vigabatrin. A number of children will relapse (have further spasms) once the steroid medication is discontinued. Relapses occur less frequently when vigabatrin is discontinued. Unfortunately steroids, and particularly the tetracosactide or ACTH which are given by intramuscular injection, may be associated with serious side-effects, and therefore the children must be monitored very closely. These side-effects include:

◆ irritability and poor sleep

◆ weight gain

◆ hypertension (high blood pressure) and occasionally heart failure

◆ diabetes mellitus

◆ susceptibility to serious infection including meningitis.

These side-effects do go away once the steroid is discontinued. Another serious side-effect of steroids is that they can reduce the body's ability to fight infections and some children may become very unwell and, rarely, may even die because of an overwhelming infection. None of these serious side-effects occur with vigabatrin. If vigabatrin is used for more than 12 months, some children may develop a problem with their peripheral vision. However, this is very unlikely to occur in children who are treated with vigabatrin for less than 6 months. One of us uses vigabatrin to treat every child who has infantile spasms, irrespective of the cause because it has so few side-effects, particularly when compared with steroids. If vigabatrin has not stopped the spasms within 10–14 days of its use, then it is always replaced with another drug, such as prednisolone. Other drugs which may be useful in treating infantile spasms (West syndrome) include sodium valproate (Epilim), nitrazepam (Mogadon) and pyridoxine. It is possible that some of the newer anti-epileptic drugs such as topiramate (Topamax), zonisamide (Zonegran) or levetiracetam (Keppra) may also be effective in some children but more research needs to be undertaken in the use of these drugs in treating West syndrome.

7

The long-term outlook

→ Key points

- Seizures eventually stop with treatment for the great majority (70 per cent) of people with epilepsy; however, some types of epilepsy are easier to control than others.

- Once seizures have stopped for 2-3 years the person with epilepsy will need to consider the pros and cons of staying on or withdrawing treatment. Around 40 per cent of those withdrawing treatment will have a seizure in the next 2 years compared to around 20 per cent of those who stay on treatment.

- It is difficult to predict precisely who will and who will not have a seizure if they withdraw treatment.

Many patients, family doctors, and even paediatricians and neurologists, can be remarkably pessimistic about the likelihood of seizures stopping; a pessimism which is unjustified by the facts. In the past, when neurologists were fewer on the ground, they tended to see only those with the worst epilepsy with the worst prognosis. As they taught the future family doctors, these too acquired the same pessimism.

What are the facts? The first point to define is what we mean by remission or cessation of seizures. Epilepsy was defined in Chapter 1 as a 'continuing tendency to epileptic seizures'. Because seizures are unpredictable recurrent events, it is difficult to give a definition of remission that everyone will agree with. Clearly, the main aim of treatment is to stop seizures, but how long should seizures have stopped for, before we say they are in remission? In research studies that have investigated the long term prognosis for populations of people with epilepsy, the absence of seizures for 5 years (a 5-year remission) is considered remission. However, the absence of seizures for shorter periods of time, such as 12 months (a 12-month remission), are also important measures as a 12-month remission will enable the person to regain their driving licence in the UK.

The best evidence about 5-year remissions from seizures comes from the work in Olmstead County, USA, to which we have already referred in Chapter 1. Figure 7.1 is redrawn from this study and shows the proportion of people whose seizures are in remission according to three definitions.

The *top curve* indicates the probability of completing a period of five consecutive years without seizures. For example, 6 years after diagnosis 42 per cent of patients have been seizure free for 5 years.

The *middle curve* is the probability of being in remission, at any time, for at least the past 5 years. The difference between the top and middle curve is due to relapse after achievement of a 5-year remission. For example at 20 years after diagnosis, 70 per cent of patients are currently free from seizures and have been for 5 years; a further 6 per cent have had at least one seizure-free period of at least 5 years' duration, but have subsequently relapsed. Data from

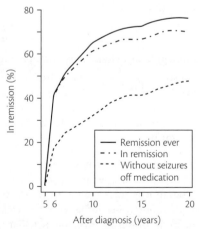

Figure 7.1 Prognosis of epilepsy; 5-year remission rates.

the National General Practice Study of Epilepsy are very similar. At 6 years after a seizure of any type (excluding acute symptomatic and single seizures) 92 per cent of people had achieved a remission lasting at least 1 year, 67 per cent lasting at least 3 years, and 42 per cent, a remission lasting at least 5 years—this last figure being identical to that from Olmstead County in the USA. The information about remission that we have considered so far includes patients continuing to take their anti-epileptic drug treatment.

Finally, the *lowest curve* indicates the probability of being free of seizures for at least 5 years whilst not taking anti-epileptic drugs; by 20 years, around half of the patients have been able to stop their treatment. Later in this chapter we discuss anti-epileptic drug withdrawal.

In summary, 20 years after diagnosis 50 per cent of patients were free from seizures without anti-epileptic drugs for at least 5 years. A further 20 per cent continue to take anti-epileptic medication and have also been free of seizures for at least 5 years. Seizures continue, in spite of medication, in 30 per cent. (Data from Dr J.F. Annegers and colleagues.)

Long-term outlook in children

It is difficult to provide an overall prognosis for epilepsy in children, because of the differing ages of onset, different epilepsy syndromes, differing causes of epilepsy, and the varying response to treatment. However, certain factors are known to be associated with a poor outcome, with seizures unresponsive or only partly responsive to treatment. These factors include:

◆ epilepsy that starts before the age of 2 or 3 years;

◆ seizure types that include myoclonic (jerk) or atonic (drop) seizures;

◆ seizures that are initially difficult to control;

◆ the need for more than one anti-epileptic drug to obtain control of the seizures;

◆ the association of other neurological problems, such as moderate or severe learning difficulties, or physical disabilities such as cerebral palsy; and

◆ if a cause has been identified (e.g. abnormal development of the brain, as in tuberous sclerosis (Chapter 3), or following meningitis or encephalitis (Chapter 3).

There are other factors which indicate a good prognosis. These include:

- epilepsy that starts after 5 but before 13 years of age;

- seizure types that include typical absence (petit mal) seizures or tonic–clonic seizures;

- ready control of seizures, using just one anti-epileptic drug;

- a lack of other associated neurological problems;

- the absence of an identified cause; and

- the presence of a strong family history of epilepsy.

Many of the epilepsies in children can be classified into epilepsy syndromes. One of the purposes of this classification is to give some guidance on the prognosis or outcome as well as the choice of treatment. Syndromes that have a poor prognosis include West syndrome (in which the seizure type is infantile spasms) and Lennox–Gastaut syndrome (seizure types include atonic, tonic, and tonic–clonic seizures). Seizures in both these syndromes start before the age of 3 years (rarely between 3 and 7 years in Lennox–Gastaut syndrome), and this in itself carries an unfavourable prognosis. Syndromes that have a good outcome include childhood absence epilepsy (petit mal) (Chapter 2) and some partial epilepsies (for example, benign partial epilepsy with centro-temporal (rolandic) spikes). In childhood absence epilepsy, between 70 and 75 per cent of children will stop having absence seizures by the age of 14–16 years and the anti-epileptic medication can be withdrawn. The remaining 25–30 per cent may need to continue taking medication into adult life, perhaps even for the rest of their lives. The children that are likely to fall into this group are those in whom absences began after the age of 11 or 12 years, were associated with generalized tonic–clonic seizures, and in whom the seizures were difficult to control.

Benign partial epilepsy with centro-temporal (rolandic) spikes is, as the name suggests, really benign. The vast majority of children with this epilepsy syndrome will have stopped having seizures by 14–16 years of age, and medication can be withdrawn with no risk of relapse (recurrence) of seizures.

Some syndromes have an intermediate outlook. One of these is juvenile myoclonic epilepsy which usually starts between 10 and 18 years of age. The seizures (myoclonic and generalized tonic–clonic) are usually easily controlled by one drug (sodium valproate), but if the medication is withdrawn, the seizures may recur. Most (but not all) patients who have this type of epilepsy will have to take the treatment for the rest of their lives.

Overall, approximately 30–40 per cent of children will outgrow their epilepsy before they become adults. This means that the anti-epileptic medication can be withdrawn. Over 70 per cent of children with typical absence epilepsy will probably be able to have their medication withdrawn after they have been seizure-free for between two and three years. In contrast, over 90 per cent of children with Lennox–Gastaut syndrome will probably need to take anti-epileptic drugs for most of their lives.

Associated neurological problems

The presence of learning difficulties or physical disabilities in association with epilepsy usually carries a poor outlook. However, this does not necessarily mean either that the epilepsy has caused the additional problems, or that these problems have been responsible for the poor outcome. What it usually means is that the underlying abnormality of the brain (of whatever cause) has been severe enough to produce both an epilepsy which is difficult to treat and other neurological problems.

Long-term outlook in adults

The factors that predict a poor outlook in adults are also well known. The first is that if the epilepsy is initially difficult to control, then it will usually continue to be difficult to control. The longer the seizures have continued, the less likely they are to stop. Other poor prognostic factors include evidence of structural brain damage, as manifest by associated neurological signs (e.g. hemiparesis— weakness on one side of the body), the occurrence of partial seizures, and the occurrence of episodes of status epilepticus. Exceptions to this general rule are that neurological signs and seizures arising as a result of strokes in older age are not generally difficult to control.

Stopping anti-epileptic medication

Children with epilepsy and their parents, and adults with epilepsy obviously want to know whether or when it is sensible to stop anti-epileptic medication once they have been free of seizures for two or three years. As Figure 7.1 shows, 20 years after diagnosis, 50 per cent of a community sample will have been free from all seizures without anti-epileptic drugs for at least five years, and many will have discontinued their drugs far earlier.

People considering withdrawing their anti-epileptic drug treatment need to consider the pros and cons of either continuing to take their treatment or withdrawing it. The pros of withdrawing treatment include the elimination of side-effects, including effects on the development of children born to women with epilepsy, and reducing the often perceived inconvenience associated with taking regular medication. The cons of withdrawing treatment include the risk of further seizures, which could have important consequences such as the loss of a driving licence for another 12 months. The best information to inform people about the risk of seizure recurrence comes from the Medical Research Council Anti-epileptic Drug Withdrawal Study undertaken in the UK, which studies people whose seizures had stopped for two or more years. One thousand people took part in this randomized study, half of whom stayed on their usual treatment and half had their treatment withdrawn. On average, after two years, 41 per cent of patients withdrawing treatment had a seizure relapse whilst 22 per cent continuing treatment had a relapse.

This study was also able to identify factors that were associated with a higher seizure relapse rate. These included:

◆ presence of myoclonic seizures, primarily those with juvenile myoclonic epilepsy

◆ the duration of time people had been free of seizures (the shorter the duration, the higher the chance of relapse)

◆ the number of anti-epileptic drugs taken

◆ whether seizures had occurred since starting treatment

◆ abnormal EEG.

Although people with an abnormal EEG are more likely to have a recurrence, it is important to emphasize that the EEG should not be thought of as a test that strongly predicts recurrence risk on its own. There will be many people with a normal EEG who go on to have further seizures, and similarly many patients with an abnormal EEG that remain free from seizures. For this reason, most specialists do not routinely organize an EEG before considering treatment withdrawal, but advise according to the type of seizure or epilepsy syndrome that the patient has, the presence of any neurological deficits and the duration or period that the patient has been seizure-free.

Once a decision has been made to withdraw anti-epileptic drug treatment, the next decision to make is the speed at which the drug should be withdrawn. There is general agreement that treatment should not be stopped abruptly, but there is little evidence to suggest the best speed of withdrawal. Most clinicians will advise treatment withdrawal over 2 to 3 months or so for most drugs. Some drugs such a phenobarbital are withdrawn more slowly, as are some of the benzodiazepines such as clonazepam and diazepam, although these drugs are not commonly used to treat epilepsy. Rarely, an anti-epileptic drug will have to be stopped more quickly (over a couple of days), and usually when the person has developed an acute allergic reaction to the drug, e.g. skin rash, swelling of the face or difficulty with their breathing.

8

Living with epilepsy

→ Key points

- When someone has a convulsion move them away from any dangerous situation where they may hurt themselves. Never try to open their mouth or put anything into it. As soon as the convulsion has stopped move them into the recovery position.

- People with epilepsy can participate in most sporting and leisure activities, such as swimming, provided sensible precautions are taken.

- Most people with epilepsy do not have seizures triggered by flashing lights (photosensitivity). People that are photosensitive should watch TV in a well-lit room and not sit too close to the TV.

- Most children with epilepsy are educated in mainstream schools, but some require special schools.

- Some occupations are not open to people with epilepsy, and people with epilepsy need appropriate careers advice. The Disability Discrimination Act and Access to Work scheme have helped people with epilepsy obtain and keep many types of employment.

- People with epilepsy are not allowed to drive in the UK unless

  - they have gone 12 months without a seizure, or

  - they have had only seizures during sleep for 3 years or more

- Anxiety and depression do occur in people with epilepsy and it is important to recognize and treat them.

What to do during a seizure

What should a bystander do during a tonic–clonic convulsion? The onset is often so sudden that it is difficult to do anything at all in the early stage, though it may be possible to break the person's fall. Parents or other relatives may recognize the warning signs that may occur if the generalized seizure follows a focal discharge, and so may have time to help the person to a chair or to a bed before the convulsion begins.

Don't try to open the person's clenched mouth, or try to put anything into their mouth. The tongue, if bitten, is bitten at the onset of the attack, so there is no point in trying to protect it. If the bystander uses his own fingers to try to force the mouth open, they may well be bitten. If he tries to force a spoon or pencil between the teeth, the person's teeth may be damaged. These manoeuvres are still sometimes attempted by tradition, and sometimes, because it is presumed that the person's blue colour and the fact that breathing has stopped are due to obstruction to the passage of air into the lungs. Attempts to 'loosen the collar' presumably result from the same thoughts. However, all of us have enough gaps between our teeth to allow passage of air around them as readers can readily show for themselves by clenching their teeth, pinching the nose, and breathing in. Obstruction to the airway may occur during, or just after, a seizure, if the person is lying on his back. The tongue may then fall backwards into the pharynx, and, for this reason, it is worth turning someone suffering a convulsion seizure into a position halfway between lying on their side and face. This is called the 'recovery position'. This position also has the advantage that if the person vomits, as occasionally happens, the contents of the stomach pass easily out of the mouth, and there is no danger of vomit entering the trachea and lungs. If a tonic–clonic seizure occurs in a public place, it usually happens that someone calls an ambulance, very often to the annoyance of the person with epilepsy, who is well on the way to recovery by the time the ambulance driver delivers him to the local hospital. There is no need to call an ambulance unless it is clear that repeated or prolonged seizures are occurring.

There is usually little to be done during a partial seizure, except to stand nearby to ensure the person is not in danger of injury. Occasionally gentle restraint may be necessary in the case of complex automatic behaviour.

Sensible restrictions on activities

Many people or relatives of people with epilepsy are naturally concerned about what may happen during a seizure if a relative or friend is not present to assist. This can be a major source of anxiety, but in reality, harm resulting from seizures is exceptionally rare. However, there are a few sensible precautions.

Children with epilepsy—what can and what can't they do?

We emphasize that a vast majority of children who have epilepsy can take part in all the activities and games that make childhood such a fun and exciting time of life. Unfortunately many people, including parents, are so afraid and concerned about what may happen if a child has an attack that they become over-protective. Being over-protective can of course be harmful in itself. It may result in the child failing to learn to do things for themselves and develop the necessary skills to become independent. This is very important because parents will not be around forever to care for their children. It is important to take a balanced view about potential risks and benefits of particular activities. For example, swimming is perfectly safe, providing it is not done alone, but with someone who knows what to do if a seizure does occur in the pool. The swimming-pool attendant must also be told. The child should not swim in deep or very cold water, and if in the sea, should never be out of their depth and be within wading distance of land. Someone should always be close to them when they are swimming in open water, such as a lake or the sea. For sailing, obviously a life-jacket should be worn.

Cycling and horse riding are popular activities, and safety helmets should always be worn by everyone who cycles or rides, whether or not they have epilepsy. Care should be taken when cycling on a busy road or in traffic, and if someone's seizures are not well-controlled then they should not cycle on a road but in a park or playground. Horse-riders should not ride alone, in case an accident takes place.

Most children enjoy climbing—whether it is trees, rocks and cliffs on the beach, or apparatus in the gym at school. Where the child's epilepsy is fully controlled, climbing is usually safe. However, when the epilepsy is poorly controlled, it is probably unwise to climb mountains (using ropes) either alone or with friends, as the risk of severe injuries (to others as well as oneself) is greater if there is a fall due to a seizure.

Sports such as badminton, squash, tennis, hockey, and football are likely to be entirely safe. It is reasonable to take part in contact sports such as rugby and wrestling, but boxing is best avoided. A very small proportion of people with epilepsy may have seizures triggered by flashing or flickering lights, particularly if they are tired. Certain precautions should be taken when playing video games or even when watching television. These include the following:

 ◆ computer screens only rarely cause seizures, and flat screen computer monitors and TVs are even less likely to trigger seizures

♦ sitting at least ten feet from the TV screen

♦ when changing TV channels use a remote control unit, or if there is no remote control, one eye should be covered as the channel is changed

♦ video games should not be played in a dark room; a bright light should be on in the room. It is best to avoid playing these at night, when tired.

Most parents of children who do not have epilepsy will encourage adventures and taking part in activities, whilst taking sensible precautions to reduce the risk of injury, even though there are always certain hazards—and accidents do happen, such as falling off bicycles, off playground equipment, or out of trees. It is important that parents do not become overly anxious or worried about these risks, just because their child has epilepsy. Some such families live in constant fear of the recurrence of a seizure—in the home, at school, or just outside playing. This fear is very easily detected by children, so that everyone becomes afraid of epilepsy and further seizures. Other parents may be ashamed of their child's epilepsy and will never talk about it. This may result in the child becoming isolated, withdrawn, and ashamed of having epilepsy, which may then limit their expectations and opportunities in life.

Education

Most children with epilepsy attend normal mainstream schools and can participate fully in the schools' curricular and extra-curricular activities. This is the case even in children in whom the epilepsy is not fully controlled. It is important for the teachers and for the school doctor and nurse to know that a child has epilepsy—even if the child's seizures are controlled. Teachers will then know what to expect and what to do if the child has a seizure. The teacher may also involve children in the class in the care of the child after a seizure; this is important for two reasons. First, it teaches children how to help someone in a seizure, and secondly—and perhaps more importantly— it shows children that there is no need to be scared or upset when someone has a fit. Hopefully, such activities may reduce, in future generations, some of the misunderstandings and social prejudice which still surround epilepsy.

About one-fifth of children with epilepsy are not able to attend a normal school. This may simply be because of different and frequent seizure types which are not fully controlled. However, the more common reason for these children not being able to attend a normal school is that they have additional problems, such as moderate or severe learning difficulties or physical disabilities (or both), in addition to their epilepsy. Most of these children will attend special schools, usually within the local neighbourhood. In this situation in the UK, under the terms of the Education Act, the child will have an assessment or statement made of his or her educational needs so that the most appropriate school can be found. This statement is based on reports from doctors (including the hospital doctor), teachers, clinical psychologists, therapists, and any other specialist who may have been involved with the child. The ultimate decision as to which school the child should attend rests with the parent.

Perhaps 1–2 per cent of all children with epilepsy may need to attend a school specifically established for children with epilepsy. These schools are usually residential or boarding schools, and the staff have special expertise in teaching children with epilepsy, in coping with their seizures, and in generally supporting them. One of the additional benefits provided by these schools is that they allow some separation from the family, which can be particularly helpful when anxiety about seizures has resulted in a degree of over-protection that has a limiting influence on the child's ability to participate in normal activities and gain a degree of independence. The environment provided by these schools encourages self-reliance.

Occasionally, a child with epilepsy, though not having frequent major seizures, may be doing badly in school. This is rarely because the child is having frequent brief seizures that have not been picked up. In this situation prolonged EEG recordings can be helpful to identify whether this is happening. Another rare possibility, but one that is often put forward, is that the child's poor school work is due to the effect of the anti-epileptic drugs. However, if the child is not excessively sleepy or drowsy, then it is most unlikely that the drugs are interfering significantly with school work. Exceptions include phenobarbital, phenytoin and topiramate, which may affect a child's concentration and therefore their learning potential, although these first two drugs are rarely used for children in the UK. In these situations the amount of drug in the blood may need to be checked. The most common reason for learning problems in a child with epilepsy is that intellectual difficulty and epilepsy share a common cause. Both are caused due to the abnormal development of the brain or brain damage (for example, after meningitis or a head injury). In these situations, an educational psychologist will assess the child's strengths and weaknesses, and recommend the most appropriate school (this is the statement of a child's educational needs mentioned earlier).

Children up until the age of 16 years are well cared for by society, educationally, and medically. The difficult time comes after the age of 16 years—the adolescent period which brings changes in social, family, and educational life. This is often a difficult time of life, even for those who do not have epilepsy. Many changes occur at adolescence which need to be coped with. Young people may find it difficult to take their anti-epileptic drug regularly, or they may deliberately decide not to do so. This is more likely to occur in teenagers who have recently been diagnosed and who may find it difficult to come to terms with the diagnosis and need for regular treatment. This may be just one part of a wider difficulty in coming to terms with having epilepsy, the need for treatment, and an increasing awareness of some of the stigma and limitations they may face, such as the inability to gain a driving licence until they have gone 12 months without a seizure. It is important that the family and the doctor explore these concerns with the teenager, are supportive, and address any misunderstandings or misconceptions.

There are a number of educational possibilities beyond the normal school-leaving age. Many young people with epilepsy will obtain higher qualifications at school and then obtain a place at college or university. It is important that college or university tutors and examiners are told about students who have epilepsy as this promotes and encourages increased awareness and understanding. Those students who live away from home in halls of residence or in rented accommodation should tell friends and college or university tutors.

Most paediatricians would not think it sensible to continue seeing patients over the age of 16 years. Teenagers of 17 or 18 years have questions and needs that reflect this transition to adult life. All too often the transfer from paediatric to adult services is poorly planned. The family doctor will continue his or her support, but consideration should be given to transferring care to a neurologist who has a special interest in epilepsy. A special clinic for teenagers with epilepsy has been established in Liverpool and other centres in the UK to ensure that there is a smooth handover of care from a children's epilepsy clinic to an adult clinic, and in which the specific issues and problems of teenagers can be dealt with satisfactorily.

Teenagers will often have chaotic sleeping patterns, and may stay up particularly late some nights. For some people, deprivation of sleep might trigger seizures, particularly those with a generalized form of epilepsy, such as juvenile myoclonic epilepsy. It is important to encourage a regular sleeping pattern, and to encourage a lie-in after a late night.

Teenagers are also exposed to, and explore, the social drinking of alcohol. An occasional drink containing alcohol is unlikely to be harmful. However, alcohol can make anti-epileptic medication less effective and may, in excess, bring on a seizure. Often, late nights and alcohol excess are combined, resulting in an increased risk of a seizure, which usually occurs in the morning the following day. It is important to get the balance right. Medical research suggests that drinking more than two units of alcohol in less than 12–15 hours may significantly increase the risk of seizures in patients who have epilepsy (2 units = one pint of beer, lager, or cider, or 2 glasses of wine, or two measures [shorts] of spirits such as whisky, rum, vodka, or gin).

Contraception will also begin to emerge as an important issue during this time. The most effective form of contraception is the pill. The oral contraceptive pill does not make epileptic seizures more or less likely to happen and there is no reason why women with epilepsy cannot take the pill. However, as has already been discussed in Chapter 6, certain anti-epileptic drugs may reduce the efficacy of the contraceptive pill, resulting in an unwanted pregnancy. A contraceptive pill with a high oestrogen content may need to be prescribed, but other forms of contraception (injection, coil, condom or cap plus spermicide) should be considered. For women taking lamotrigine when the pill is started, the dose of lamotrigine might need to be increased.

Prejudice, and telling others about epilepsy

It is unfortunately true that those with epilepsy do encounter a fair amount of prejudice against them, especially in the field of employment (Chapter 5). This prejudice is probably largely due to ignorance. As discussed in Chapter 1, there is folklore around epilepsy which may be perceived to be associated with mental illness, learning difficulties, and other problems, which may limit the expectations of an employer, even if the person with epilepsy does not have any of these associated problems. Similarly, fear can also be a major factor, as employers and colleagues may be frightened of having to deal with someone having a seizure, which may not be something that they have done before. A major decision that someone with epilepsy has to make, therefore, is how much to tell, and to whom. This will depend on the circumstances and the degree of control of the epilepsy.

Young people with epilepsy forming friendships with the opposite sex also suffer agonies about these decisions. If the epilepsy is not talked about early in the relationship the subject becomes more and more difficult to bring up. The problem may then be revealed by the occurrence of a seizure without prior explanation. Both parties feel devastated, the one guilty and ashamed at not having had the courage to explain the problem, the other surprised and ashamed of their surprise and inability to cope both with the seizure and their own feelings about it. On balance, we are sure that it is best for a person with epilepsy to tell those he meets frequently something of the facts, so that they can cope with a seizure if it occurs. Friends will appreciate the confidence shown in them by the disclosure of this fact.

Psychological and psychiatric disorders and epilepsy

People with epilepsy have to cope with the effects of their seizures on their chances in life—which may well be reduced if seizures are frequent. Their circle of friends and choice of sexual partner may well be narrowed down. Their inability to hold a driving licence and limitations in employment reduce their earning power, social status, and long-term financial security. By avoidance of factors which they believe may precipitate seizures, social activities may be greatly reduced. It is not surprising, therefore, that people with epilepsy become anxious, or depressed, or resentful, and irritable.

The age of onset of epilepsy may also influence the psychological effects suffered. A man of 45 in previous good health who then develops epilepsy is likely to have already established his personality, social life, family, and career. Although he may have problems with future employment, there will probably be no change in how his friends and family perceive him and react to him. However, it may be different for a girl whose epilepsy begins at the age of 14 or 15, with frequent seizures throughout her school career, who might have fewer educational, employment, and social opportunities. Although both may become anxious or depressed, this is probably more likely to happen in the teenage girl.

It is important the anxiety and depression are picked up as they usually improve with appropriate treatment. The GP and neurologist should enquire about anxiety and depression at appointments, because symptoms of anxiety and depression are not always sought and thus can go untreated for significant lengths of time. There are a number of approaches to treatment which include psychological methods such as cognitive behavioural treatment or counselling, and drug treatments. Doctors with limited experience of treating depression in people with epilepsy are often concerned that the antidepressant drugs might trigger seizures. The risk of this is actually very small, and if the depression requires drug treatment, then this should usually be given.

A psychotic illness with symptoms similar to those of paranoid schizophrenia may occasionally be seen in those with epilepsy arising from a temporal lobe lesion. The occurrence of the psychosis is not necessarily related to the frequency of seizures. Indeed, there is an interesting group of patients in whom the psychosis becomes prominent as seizures come under control, only to remit as seizures return.

Problems for women with epilepsy

Problems facing women with epilepsy have been referred to at various places within the book. The effect of menstruation on seizure frequency is discussed in Chapter 3. The interaction between anti-epileptic drugs and oral contraceptives is discussed in Chapter 6. The effects of anti-epileptic drugs on the foetus are also discussed in Chapter 6.

Some women report that their seizures become more frequent, others less frequent during pregnancy, and others have seizures which remain more or less unchanged in pregnancy. There seems to be no way of predicting what is going to happen in the first pregnancy. By and large, subsequent pregnancies in any mother follow much the same pattern. Although epilepsy may start for the first time during pregnancy, this usually seems to be coincidental, and there is no good evidence that pregnancy itself is a cause of epilepsy. For women taking lamotrigine, it is important to understand that the levels in the blood drop in the third trimester and the dose may need to be increased. Many mothers on anti-epileptic drugs wonder whether they can breastfeed their babies. Careful studies have been made on this important issue and although varying amounts of the drugs are secreted into breast milk, this is unlikely to have any effect on the baby. If the mother is taking lamotrigine, there is a small theoretical risk that the baby might develop an allergic response to this anti-epileptic drug. If the mother is taking phenobarbital, primidone or ethosuximide, this might make her baby irritable or sleepy, and might also interfere with their feeding pattern. However, it should be emphasized that for most mothers, and most anti-epileptic drugs, it is safe for them to breastfeed their babies. The benefits and possible risks of breast feeding should always be discussed with the epilepsy specialist.

Sexual activity and epilepsy

Seizures during or immediately after intercourse are exceptionally uncommon. There is usually no reason for avoiding intercourse on the grounds that seizures may be provoked. People with epilepsy can experience problems with lack of libido and some men might find difficulty initiating or sustaining erections. The cause of these difficulties includes anxiety or depression, the epilepsy itself, and drug(s) taken for epilepsy. When these problems occur it is important for the doctor to try and identify the most likely cause and consider what can be done to help.

Employment

It is not sensible to be a window-cleaner or scaffolder if one has many seizures. But just what restrictions on employment should be applied to those with epilepsy? The 'Access to Work' scheme may provide helpful and practical advice for which jobs and type of employment may be particularly suitable.

First of all, there are the legal restrictions on driving, which are fully discussed on pp. 139–43. This may stop employment as a travelling representative, for example, but these regulations have a wider effect in making travel to a job more difficult, especially in rural areas, however suitable that job may be.

There are a number of other occupations where someone having a seizure might put themselves or others at unacceptable risks. For example, occupations where one has responsibility for other people such as surgery and nursing. This does not mean that people with epilepsy may not train for these professions, but once trained the types of responsibilities may be limited. Other occupations that are not accessible to people with epilepsy include airline pilot, train driver, railway signalman, and merchant navy sailor, etc. The armed forces, fire, and ambulance services and police also exclude those with continuing seizures.

In other jobs, there is no real risk to bystanders during a seizure, but there is a substantial risk of injury or death to the person with continuing epilepsy. The operation of heavy moving machinery, including agricultural machinery, work near conveyor belts, work at heights, particularly in the construction or electric power industries, and work underground or underwater should all be avoided. However keen the subject may be to take his own life in his hands, it is not fair to burden employers if there is a substantial risk of a mutilating or fatal accident.

One of the sometimes difficult questions that people with infrequent seizures must ask themselves is whether to tell a potential employer about them. Obviously, it is best if they do because the employer can take into account any remote risks about which the applicant is unaware. Employers can make an occasional allowance for rare but unexpected absences from work, and they can, in an informed way, cope with occasional seizures at work. The truth of the matter is that many employers reject those who have seizures that are few and far between, or those who have had no seizures for some years, for jobs which carry virtually no risk to the person with epilepsy or to others. Fortunately the introduction of the Disability Discrimination Act has been very helpful in making it much easier for someone with epilepsy to obtain employment and to protect them in their workplace if their seizures are not well-controlled.

Whatever the decision about disclosure, applicants for a job will be more successful if they follow the general rules of taking care while writing their application, taking trouble to inform themselves about the responsibilities of the post and about the employer, presenting themselves well at interviews, selling their ability to do the job, and convincing the prospective employer that they have an enthusiastic desire to work.

Obtaining a job is obviously only the first step. Most of us want promotion up to the limits of our energies and capabilities, and here again epilepsy, even if well controlled, might reduce chances in life. It is difficult to measure the frequency with which those well qualified for promotion are overlooked, but one study found that the rate of dismissal following the onset of epilepsy was increased approximately sixfold.

There is another more subtle way in which epilepsy can hinder employment and promotion. The fear of encountering rejection or the fear of leaving an established position with a tolerant employer may cause the people with epilepsy to deny themselves chances for betterment. Just as the employer may be prejudiced against people with epilepsy so may the person with epilepsy be prejudiced against employers, believing them all to be lacking in understanding.

Driving and epilepsy

There are few aspects of having epilepsy in adult life that cause greater distress than the necessary legal restrictions on driving. For those living in rural areas where public transport is limited or non-existent, car ownership and driving are necessary for shopping and social contact, and for getting to work. There are jobs such as that of a delivery van driver in which driving is the sole function of employment, and any restriction on driving will cause the employee to lose his job.

This book may well be read in a number of countries, and the legal requirements vary from place to place. As an example, however, we consider the UK eligibility to hold a private (Group 1) driving licence in the UK, which states that

> An applicant for a licence suffering from epilepsy shall satisfy the following conditions, namely that he shall
>
> a) have been free from any epileptic attack during the period of one year immediately preceding the date when the licence is granted; or

b) have had an epileptic attack whilst asleep more than three years before the date when the licence is granted and shall have had attacks only whilst asleep between the date of that attack and the date when the licence is granted; and that

c) the driving of a vehicle by him in accordance with the licence is not likely to be a danger to the public.

The purpose of clause (b) is to allow someone to drive who has established a long history of seizures whilst asleep without ever having had any whilst awake.

These Regulations are, we believe, a reasonable attempt to protect the public from the chances of meeting a driver who is briefly incapable of controlling his car because of a seizure. The Regulations are also fair to those with epilepsy insofar as they clearly state the circumstances under which they can drive without fear of causing harm to themselves or others.

What actually happens in practice? Take the example of a woman who has held a licence for several years, and then has two tonic–clonic seizures at work within a month. Her family doctor or neurologist will explain that she is no longer eligible to hold a driving licence. It is not the responsibility of either doctor to inform the licensing authority of this, but a doctor will record in their notes the fact that they have explained the position to the patient. It is the driver's responsibility to take action. Inside each UK Driving Licence is the statement that the 'Drivers Medical Branch, Swansea MUST be told at once if: you NOW have any physical or mental disability which affects your fitness as a driver or which might do so IN THE FUTURE'. The patient should write a brief note to the Driver and Vehicle Licensing Agency (DVLA) at Swansea explaining the details and enclosing the licence, which will be acknowledged. No further action is necessary. Although it is the driver's responsibility to inform the Driver and Vehicle Licensing Agency about their epilepsy, their doctor also has a duty to report their patient to the driving agency if they believe they are continuing to drive and could put other's safety at risk.

If all goes well for this woman, and she has no further seizures after the first two, she becomes eligible to hold a driving licence one year after the date of the last attack. She then completes an application form as usual.

All this seems entirely straightforward, but we know that many people with epilepsy find the Regulations hard to accept. Doctors appreciate the difficulties that may be caused by giving up driving. Driving is usually an essential part of their work, so they do not have to make great leaps of imagination to realize the difficulties that a ban on driving may cause. Unfortunately the law does not take hardship into account. Doctors should, however, not only advise their patients of the law, but also, from their experience, advise patients how to cope with their changed circumstances. Doctors are in a position to influence decisions of employers about the nature of their patients' work. They can write to the employer, with the patient's consent, supporting a request for a change of job within the same company. In such a letter, a doctor does not necessarily have to say that the person has epilepsy, only that they are not able to drive for medical reasons, and are not likely to be able to drive for some time. Such letters may well influence the company's decision. Doctors should also advise their patients about the 'Access to Work' scheme which was established to help those with a disability, including poorly controlled epilepsy. Specific advice on suitable types of work can be obtained from the Disability Employment Adviser at Jobcentre Plus Offices.

We usually advise people living in rural areas not to move house just because of their new inability to drive. If it seems likely that the seizures can be easily controlled, then it is probably better to cope somehow for the time necessary, rather than disturb the whole family's way of life. People with epilepsy are the only ones who can decide whether to move, but their doctors should give them sufficient information about the probability of seizure control to allow an informed decision.

Sometimes people with epilepsy will say that they consider it safe to drive as they always get a warning of their attacks. The fact that they are having seizures means that by law they are ineligible to drive, even in the rare case that the warning is long enough to allow them to stop the car. Similarly, the law does not distinguish between seizure types. Thus someone that is having simple partial seizures (auras) may be completely aware during the seizure, but remains ineligible by law to drive.

Another common question is about the timing of seizures. With the exception of seizures which have always occurred during sleep, the time of seizure is irrelevant. If the patient always has their seizures first thing in the morning or in the evening whilst awake, they remain ineligible to drive even if they propose to avoid driving at those times.

Sometimes a patient may feel that the events which have led him to the doctor are not epileptic seizures. All a doctor can do in such circumstances is to disagree, and advise that the patient seeks a further opinion. As noted above, it is not a doctor's responsibility to inform the licensing agency of a person's epilepsy. It may be, however, that if a doctor is convinced of the diagnosis, and believes that there is a real risk to the public, and if the patient refuses to seek a further opinion, he or she may feel that responsibility to the public at large overrides responsibility to the individual patient. It is also important to highlight that those who knowingly drive when ineligible must realize that their insurance policies would almost certainly be void if they had an accident. But the terrible risk of killing or maiming themselves or another road user or pedestrian should be sufficient discouragement.

There are no restrictions—other than those of common-sense—on riding a pedal bicycle. Even if a rider has a seizure, they are likely to damage only themselves.

The Regulations state nothing about anti-epileptic medication. The law is, as it were, interested in seizures and not in drugs. This means that there is no need to withdraw medication after a seizure-free interval so that the patient can resume driving. On common-sense grounds, it is probably marginally safer to be a passenger with someone who has had seizures in the past, who remains on anti-epileptic medication, rather than travel with someone who had his last seizure three years ago and stopped his drugs yesterday.

The Department of Health has an Honorary Medical Advisory Panel that considers specific questions about epilepsy and fitness to drive. The questions are usually over the diagnosis of epilepsy, and whether the doctor has made a correct diagnosis. This can occasionally happen with someone who has had just a single convulsion at the time of a head injury (called a concussive convulsion), or someone who has had episodes of flashing lights and tingling in an arm or leg (which occurs in migraine). Neither of these individuals should be diagnosed as having epilepsy but this may occasionally happen. Any applicant who disagrees with the Department's refusal to grant him a licence, on the grounds that he has epilepsy and does not satisfy the requirements of the Regulations, may appeal to the Advisory Panel. From a compilation of the advice given by members of the Panel, a set of guidelines has been drawn up by the Medical Officers of the Department of Transport. If there is doubt in their minds, the matter is referred to the appropriate specialist. However, it must be stated that appeals are only likely to be successful if it can be proven that the individual does not have epilepsy as in the two examples described above.

The graph shown in Chapter 7 indicates that even if a remission of seizures lasting five years has occurred, relapses do unfortunately occur. The relapse rate in the first five years after achieving a remission of five years was around 8 per cent. A study organized by the Medical Research Council in the UK has found that about a third of those who stop treatment on medical advice will have a further attack at some time, and of those about a half will have a recurrence within a year. Many will therefore consider it an additional safeguard to continue anti-epileptic medication, if driving, even if they are free from attacks. However, in the same study a number of people had attacks even though they were continuing anti-epileptic drugs so that they could be compared with those who stopped them.

Regulations for those who wish to drive heavy goods vehicles are even more strict. The current regulations state that all of the following criteria must be met. The person should have been free from epileptic attacks for 10 years, have not taken anti-epileptic medication during this 10-year period, and does not have a continuing liability to an epileptic seizure.

Finally, before we end the issue of driving, we should add two further points. So far, we have written exclusively about the practice in the UK. The requirements for eligibility vary from country to country, and, in the USA, from state to state. Enquiry must be made of the licensing authority in each country or state in which patients wish to drive.

Life insurance

One of the few ways that an average person has of building capital throughout his lifetime is by house purchase, and by payments into regular saving schemes. Couples will also usually wish to provide some sort of monetary support to their surviving partner or children in the event of unexpected early death. In short, life insurance is now regarded as part of nearly everyone's everyday financial arrangements.

Life insurance companies are in business with the primary aim of providing a financial return for their shareholders, or, in the case of a mutual office, of providing a fair deal for all policy-holders. It has to be admitted that on average the mortality of those with seizures is higher than the general population. It is therefore not surprising that the life offices, if they accept the risk of underwriting the lives of those with epilepsy, require an excess premium to compensate them for the excess risk. There is often a considerable difference between the excess rates quoted by various offices, so it is well worth seeking professional advice from an insurance broker. It is important to be honest and declare the epilepsy. If the epilepsy is not disclosed it is highly likely that the insurance company would not pay out should the person with epilepsy die. Advice on both life and travel insurance, and which are the best and most helpful firms to contact can be obtained from Epilepsy Action or the National Society for Epilepsy, whose contact details can be found at the end of this book.

Special care for those with the worst epilepsy

Most people with frequent seizures are looked after at home by devoted parents or partners. Sometimes a fragile situation breaks down and it is clear that a person with epilepsy cannot cope at home. Obviously, if it is believed that this is a purely temporary setback likely to be improved by modification of anti-epileptic medication, then the family doctor will arrange a short stay in a hospital or other appropriate unit. Occasionally, however, it is obvious that neither the domestic situation of the person with epilepsy, nor their epilepsy, is going to improve in the foreseeable future, and long-stay care has to be arranged. The precipitating factor is very often the illness or death of the last surviving supporting relative.

In the middle of the last century, an increasing social commitment to those less fortunate than the majority resulted in the establishment of a very small number of 'colonies' for people with epilepsy. The general plan of such colonies in Europe was of a totally self-contained institution. During the day, the people with epilepsy would work in the open air, in farms and gardens, and at night they would return to dormitories, or, in the more advanced colonies, to small houses in which some semblance of a family circle was maintained. Many people with severe epilepsy spent the greater part of their lives in these institutions. Happily in the UK, these colonies no longer exist. Most people with severe epilepsy are now very well-supported in the community, but there is still a need for long-term care in specialized centres for a small minority of people with epilepsy, the majority of whom have other problems including learning and physical disabilities. These specialized centres provide a wide range of high-quality diagnostic and treatment services, as well as offering safe and supervised long-term accommodation.

9

Convulsions associated with fever

➔ Key points

◆ About 1 in every 25–30 children aged 1 to 5 years will experience at least one febrile convulsion (seizure). Why only a small proportion of children who have a high temperature (called a fever or pyrexia) will then have a febrile convulsion is unclear but this is almost certainly related to genetic factors.

◆ About 1 in 3 children who have had a first febrile convulsion will go on to have a second febrile convulsion.

◆ Febrile seizures can be divided into simple and complex febrile convulsions; most febrile convulsions are simple.

◆ Complex febrile convulsions—those that are usually prolonged or affecting only one side of the body—are associated with a significantly increased risk of developing later afebrile seizures, that is, epilepsy. In these individuals, the epilepsy that develops usually arises from one of the temporal lobes.

◆ It is always important to consider an underlying cause of what appears to be a febrile convulsion in a child aged 1 year or less; specifically meningitis, encephalitis, a biochemical or genetic disorder or an abnormality in the brain.

◆ There is no indication to use an anti-epileptic drug to try and prevent further febrile convulsions or the later development of epilepsy.

◆ Buccal midazolam or rectal diazepam may be used in those children who seem to have frequent febrile convulsions and when the convulsion lasts longer than 5 or 6 minutes and shows no signs of stopping.

A convulsion that occurs in association with any illness, usually an infection, which causes a rise in temperature (called a fever or pyrexia), is known as a febrile convulsion. Febrile convulsions are also known as febrile seizures.

Febrile convulsions are not a type of epilepsy. In the past it was thought that febrile convulsions could lead to epilepsy but this is now generally believed to be only rarely the case. There are at least three subgroups of febrile convulsions:

◆ The first and largest subgroup is made up of children who have seizures in response to fever as a result of an individual susceptibility that is usually inherited. These children develop normally, have normal EEGs and normal brain scans. This is the group which constitutes 'true' febrile convulsions and will be discussed in detail later in this chapter.

◆ The second subgroup comprises children in whom the fever or high temperature acts as a trigger that unmasks epilepsy. In these children, seizures or fits *without* a high temperature or fever soon develop and these children can then be considered as having definite epilepsy. Magnetic resonance imaging (MRI) scans in these children may show an abnormality, usually in one temporal lobe (Chapter 5). However, sometimes this abnormality is not seen for some years after the child has started having epileptic seizures. Before their first febrile convulsion, many of these children may have been developing more slowly than most children—which suggests that they might have an underlying problem.

◆ The third is a very small subgroup which comprises children who convulse with fever due to meningitis or encephalitis—meaning, respectively, an inflammation or infection of the membranes covering the brain; or of the brain substance itself. Obviously it is critically important to recognize this subgroup so that antibiotic or anti-viral treatment can be started as soon as possible to treat the meningitis or encephalitis.

True febrile convulsions, as defined in the first category above, are common: 2–4 per cent of children between the ages of 6 months and 5 years will have at least one febrile convulsion. The most common age is between 12 and 20 months. It is important to be careful about accepting a diagnosis of a true febrile convulsion in a child aged less than 6 months or older than 5 years. Children aged 6 months are more likely to have meningitis or encephalitis, and children aged 6 months (or less) or 5 years (and above) are more likely to have epilepsy triggered by fever. Girls are more likely than boys to have a febrile convulsion. Up to one-third of children who have had one febrile convulsion, will go on to have a second febrile convulsion before the age of 5 years.

Most of the convulsions are tonic–clonic in type and last less than 3 or 4 minutes. This type of febrile convulsion is called simple. Complex (sometimes called 'complicated') febrile convulsions are the ones that:

◆ involve only one side of the body,

◆ last longer than 15 minutes,

◆ are followed by weakness or loss of use of one side of the body.

These complex febrile convulsions are uncommon and account for no more than 10-20 per cent (ie: a minority) of all true febrile convulsions. Complex febrile convulsions are more commonly seen in children in the other two groups described above.

Causes of febrile convulsions

The cause of a febrile convulsion is, as the name implies, a fever or high temperature. Any of the common childhood infections such as an upper respiratory, ear, bowel or urinary tract infection, chickenpox or tonsillitis may cause a high temperature and therefore cause a febrile convulsion. It is unclear whether it is how quickly the temperature rises, or how high it eventually gets that determines whether a convulsion will occur. Many children between 6 months and 5 years of age have febrile illnesses but obviously, the majority will not have a convulsion. One of the reasons why some children do, and others do not have convulsions with fever, is because of inherited factors which are important in determining whether febrile convulsions will occur. As yet it is not known what exactly these inherited factors are, but research is likely to answer this question in the next few years. Almost one-third of children will be found to have a family history of febrile convulsions in their parents or siblings (brothers and sisters):

◆ when one parent has a history of febrile convulsions, the risk to a child of developing a febrile convulsion is almost 20 per cent

◆ if both parents have a history of febrile seizures, then the risk is increased to 50 per cent

◆ the brothers and sisters of a child who has had a febrile convulsion have a three times increased risk of having a febrile convulsion themselves; this risk is even higher in identical twins.

Most children who have febrile convulsions do not need any tests. Usually, the cause of the infection and of the fever is obvious from the examination carried out by the doctor—for example, a sore throat (tonsillitis), red ear (otitis media), rash (for example, chickenpox), cold and cough, or gastroenteritis (diarrhoea and vomiting). A urinary tract infection may not be that easy to recognize by examining; the child can only really be diagnosed by testing a specimen of urine. Rarely, however, and particularly in children under 18 months of age, a convulsion may be the first sign of meningitis or encephalitis. Sometimes, a complex febrile seizure may be the first sign that a child may be about to develop a specific epilepsy syndrome called severe myoclonic epilepsy of infancy (also called Dravet syndrome). Finally, and very rarely, a complex febrile convulsion may be the first sign of an underlying biochemical (or metabolic) or genetic disorder. Usually these children have additional features including:

◆ developmental delay

◆ a small or large head

◆ poor weight gain or poor growth, or both

◆ additional abnormalities on physical examination

If there is any doubt as to whether a child may have meningitis (particularly in children aged 6–18 months), then a lumbar puncture must be done, and other tests may be required, depending on the overall condition of the child. Children with simple febrile convulsions do not need to have an EEG or brain scan. However, children with complex febrile convulsions may well need an EEG and MRI scan to see whether there is a structural abnormality in their brain to explain their prolonged or asymmetrical convulsion or earlier slow development.

Treatment

The aims of treatment of febrile convulsion are threefold:

◆ to stop the convulsion

◆ to identify and treat any underlying infection (e.g. urinary tract infection, otitis media) which might have caused the fever

◆ to try and prevent further febrile convulsions.

Febrile convulsions in most children stop of their own accord, usually after 3 or 4 minutes. Such short-lived febrile convulsions are not dangerous, do not cause brain damage and are not life-threatening.

However, if a child convulses for more than 10 minutes, and the convulsion shows no signs of stopping, then a doctor *must* be called immediately, or the child must be taken to the accident and emergency department of the nearest hospital.

It is important to try and stop a convulsion, as there is a risk that prolonged febrile convulsions, lasting more than 30 minutes, may contribute to the later development of epilepsy. In order to stop a febrile convulsion that has been lasting for more than 10 minutes, a doctor or paramedic ambulance crew may give a medicine called midazolam (also called Epistatus or Hypnovel) or diazepam (also called Valium or Stesolid). Midazolam is usually inserted into the buccal (cheek) cavity and diazepam is usually given into the rectum or injected into a vein.

Some children who have had a first febrile convulsion will be admitted to hospital for observation and to find a cause of any underlying infection. Antibiotics may be given if an infection is found. A brief admission in hospital may help to relieve parental anxiety. This is important because interviews have revealed that the parents of at least half of the children who have their first febrile convulsion believe that their child is about to die, or has in fact died.

It is very important to understand this concern and anxiety. It is also important to explain that this almost never happens and reassure that children almost always make a full recovery following a simple febrile convulsion.

About one-third of children will have a second or even third febrile convulsion. The risk of a child having a second or third febrile convulsion is greater if:

- the child is aged less than 12 months (and particularly if a girl)

- if the *first* febrile convulsion lasted more than 15–20 minutes or involved only one side of the body (i.e. was a complex febrile convulsion);

◆ if the parents or brother or sister has had febrile convulsions, or has epilepsy.

There are some simple measures which can be taken to prevent further or recurrent febrile seizures. These measures include (whenever a child has an infection and is showing a rise in temperature):

◆ undressing the child

◆ sponging him or her with tepid (lukewarm) water; **the water must not be cold because this could actually increase the risk of having a febrile convulsion**

◆ giving regular paracetamol (Calpol) or ibuprofen (Brufen) (every 3–4 hours) which brings down the temperature. **Aspirin should not be used for this purpose in very young children, as this drug may cause very serious problems in the liver.**

There are a number of situations in which a parent might predict—or expect—that the child's temperature may well increase, and therefore, that a febrile convulsion *may* occur. Such a situation might be after an immunization or vaccination (for example, the triple vaccine, given three times in the first year of life, or the MMR—mumps, measles, rubella—vaccine given between 15 and 18 months of age). It is quite safe and sensible to give paracetamol at the time of vaccination and for 24–48 hours afterwards. With the MMR vaccine, there may be a very mild measles-like illness (with a high fever) 8–10 days after the vaccine has been given, and again, it would be wise to anticipate this rise in the child's temperature and give paracetamol or ibuprofen around that time.

In the past, anti-epileptic drugs were used to try and prevent further febrile convulsions from happening:

◆ it was shown that sodium valproate (Epilim) and phenytoin (Epanutin) were unsuccessful in preventing further febrile convulsions, and also did not alter the occurrence of convulsions without fever—that is, it does not prevent epileptic seizures from developing in later childhood

◆ although phenobarbital has been shown to be effective in a few children, this drug may cause significant side-effects in young children and therefore doctors do not recommend using this medication to try and prevent further febrile convulsions.

In those few children who have repeated or long febrile convulsions, midazolam (Epistatus or Hypnovel) may be given bucally or diazepam (Valium, Stesolid) may be given rectally, by parents after appropriate training. This medicine is used to prevent or stop any convulsion that has lasted more than 5 or 6 minutes and shows no signs of stopping. Fortunately, it is only rarely necessary to prescribe this medication for children with febrile convulsions.

Outcome of children with febrile convulsions

A number of population-based studies have been undertaken in both Great Britain and the United States of America that have assessed the outcome of children who have experienced febrile convulsions. In one large prospective study of over 50,000 children carried out by the National Institute of Neurological and Communicative Disorders and Strokes in the USA, the incidence of febrile convulsions was about 3 per cent, and the recurrence rate 32 per cent. By the time that the children had reached the age of 7 years, more than one non-febrile seizure (that is, an epileptic seizure) had developed in 0.5 per cent of those who had *never* had a febrile convulsion, and in four times as many, 2 per cent, of these who *had* a febrile convulsion. Children who had experienced a complex (i.e. prolonged or focal) febrile convulsion, and who also had evidence of pre-existing developmental delay, were eight times more likely to develop epilepsy by the age of 7 years than children with simple febrile convulsions, and 18 times more likely than children who had never had a febrile convulsion at all. These figures show that one cannot completely ignore the relationship or association between some febrile convulsions (the complex febrile seizures) and epilepsy. In summary:

◆ For those children who have had two or more complex febrile seizures (particularly prolonged febrile seizures lasting 15 minutes or more) and who also have developmental delay, the risk of developing epilepsy later is considerably higher, approximately 20–25 per cent.

◆ However, the parents of a child who have had one or only two simple febrile convulsions and who have shown a normal development and who have a normal neurological examination, can be assured that the chances of epilepsy developing subsequently are very low—only between 1 and 2 per cent—and that their child has about 98 chances out of 100 of not developing non-febrile, epileptic seizures. This is the very important take-home message.

10

The future: hope or hype?

There is no doubt that the understanding and treatment of epilepsy has improved considerably over the past twenty years and particularly over the past decade. Improvement has been obvious in the following areas:

- basic, laboratory-based, scientific research, which has given new insights into understanding how and why epilepsy occurs and how epilepsy may be related to a group of disorders called channelopathies

- the genetics, or inheritance, of epilepsy and the recognition that many epilepsies have a genetic basis, although the genetics is still very complex

- the development of drugs that are targeted against the precise causes of seizures, including the channels through which the chemicals and neuro-transmitters pass that are responsible for causing the seizures

- the development of more effective, but more importantly, safer anti-epileptic drugs by the pharmaceutical industry

- the consideration of performing a surgical procedure sooner rather than later

- the establishment of epilepsy nurses, which are becoming as common as diabetes nurses. It is now recognized that epilepsy nurses, together with adequately trained and experienced doctors in epilepsy, are equally important in providing a hospital-based epilepsy clinic or epilepsy service

- the beginning of new research into whether epilepsy might be prevented following severe head injuries and following meningitis and encephalitis

- a continuing reduction in the stigma of epilepsy—at school, in the work place and in the community

Despite these advances, there is still a huge amount of research and work that needs to be undertaken, not only to improve our understanding and knowledge, but to improve the quality of life of every child or man or woman with epilepsy.

> Unfortunately, despite these advances, it remains very unlikely that a single treatment (anti-epileptic drug, operation or completely new type of treatment) or 'cure' for all epileptic seizures and epilepsies will ever be found, due to the fact that there are so many different types of epileptic seizure and epilepsy syndromes and also many different causes of epilepsy.

It is also very unlikely that most of the epilepsies will ever be completely prevented from occurring in the first place—although this is an area which has been poorly researched in the past and, in the authors' opinion, should be much more actively researched in the future. Although a significant proportion of the epilepsies are inherited, it is unlikely that much can be done to prevent these epilepsies, and it may not be possible (or appropriate) to remove these abnormal genes by genetic engineering techniques. However, if the epilepsy occurs as a part of a progressive condition, as in the group of conditions called Batten's disease (Chapter 5), it is possible that epilepsy might be prevented if the abnormal gene causing these conditions could be switched-off. Improved medical care could—and, more importantly, should—reduce the number of individuals who develop epilepsy following premature birth or birth asphyxia, meningitis or encephalitis. Improved safety measures on the roads, in cars, the possible raising of the legal age at which people can drive to 18 or 19 years of age, a considerable tightening of drink-drive laws (zero tolerance) and the wider use of cycle helmets and protective head gear on industrial sites should reduce the incidence of post-traumatic epilepsy. In developing countries, better obstetric care and public health measures to eradicate parasitic diseases (particularly cysticercosis and malaria) and bacterial diseases (particularly tuberculosis and other causes of meningitis) will also be important in reducing the incidence (the number of new cases per year) and therefore the prevalence of epilepsy.

Medication

New drugs

In the past many new drugs were tested on their ability to stop experimental seizures in animals, usually rats and mice. This is how the drugs phenobarbitone (also called phenobarbital), phenytoin, carbamazepine, and sodium valproate were discovered. However, because such a drug's action is not just on stopping seizures, other effects, some unwanted and unpleasant, are common. Biochemical and neurological research has identified many chemicals (including neurotransmitters) which have helped to explain how and why seizures may start (and stop). One of the most important of these neurotransmitters has been, and remains, gamma aminobutyric acid (GABA), which acts by inhibiting or stopping seizures. Knowing this information has led to research which has tried to develop designer drugs which target or directly affect these neurotransmitters. The first of these was vigabatrin, which, by increasing the concentration of GABA within the brain, prevents seizures from happening. Other neurotransmitters called glutamate and aspartate have the opposite effect to GABA and can stimulate, rather than inhibit a seizure, or make a seizure more likely to happen. Lamotrigine and topiramate are drugs that were partially designed to reduce the effect of these excitatory neurotransmitters in the brain and therefore prevent seizures. Unfortunately, it has not been that straightforward to find other designer drugs, mainly because the brain is a very complex organ, including the extremely complex interaction of its very many neurotransmitters. Nevertheless, considerable research continues to try and find not just more effective anti-epileptic drugs, but safer ones with less unwanted side-effects and also ones that may only have to be given once a day. Giving drugs just once a day reduces the chance that someone will forget to take a dose; reduces the nuisance or hassle of having to take medication twice a day, and therefore improves compliance. This is particularly important for the teenager and the young adult.

Pharmaco-resistance

A great deal of research is currently being undertaken to try and understand why individuals with the same type of seizures and the same type of epilepsy show completely different responses to the same dose of anti-epileptic drug. This is known as pharmaco-resistance, which means literally a lack of, or poor response to anti-epileptic drugs. It is almost certain that pharmaco-resistance is common and that it has a genetic basis. The challenge for researchers is to translate any new information and understanding of pharmaco-resistance into improved treatment of people with epilepsy; unfortunately, as with most genetic advances, this is likely to be easier said than done.

Surgery

Without doubt, surgical treatment of epilepsy will continue to increase over the next decade. This is because brain scanning and EEG techniques will become even more advanced, and more widely available, thereby enabling the identification of subtle abnormalities within the brain responsible for seizures, some of which will be capable of being removed surgically. A greater understanding and use of brain scanning investigations should be particularly helpful, including:

◆ magneto-electroencephalography (MEG)

◆ functional MRI (fMRI)

◆ MRI tractography

◆ brand new ways of looking at how exactly the brain functions.

These investigations will also help the neurologists and neurosurgeons to reduce the occurrence of any unwanted effects of surgery. What will become increasingly important is that epilepsy surgery will be undertaken earlier and earlier, including in infants and young children. This will hopefully reduce the burden of frequent seizures with its consequent adverse effect on a child's or young person's education and employment—and also reduce the anxieties and suffering of the child's family. However, to fulfil this hope and expectation there will have to be an expansion in the number of specialist centres that can undertake the detailed assessment of children and people with epilepsy, and then safely perform the appropriate surgical procedures. At the current time, there is huge deficiency of these epilepsy centres, not just in the UK, but throughout the rest of Europe. Despite these advances, and to emphasize what was discussed in Chapter 6, it will continue to be likely that only a relatively small number of all patients (perhaps no more than 10–15 per cent) will ever be suitable for surgical treatment.

Quality of life of children and people with epilepsy

Over the past decade, there has been an increased attempt to consider and take into account the opinions and feelings of people with epilepsy and their families. This includes asking about and assessing the effect of epilepsy on aspects of their life such as choice of career, employment, social and leisure activities, and family life. Collectively, these assessments are known as 'quality of life' assessments and have focused on a person's life and not just how frequently their seizures occur. It is still true that epilepsy carries a stigma and consequently some prejudice, and it remains true that the relatively poor medical understanding and management of epilepsy has contributed to patients with epilepsy experiencing a relatively poor quality of life. Fortunately, both the stigma from having epilepsy and the prejudice against people with epilepsy is diminishing, and this is for many reasons:

- an increased understanding about how epilepsy is caused

- an increased medical awareness of the condition at all levels of undergraduate and postgraduate medical training

- the development of more effective and safer drugs, and of surgical treatments leading to improved control of seizures

- the development of specialist epilepsy clinics and facilities, both locally in general hospitals and nationally in major specialist centres

- the appointment of nurses in epilepsy whose role is to support and counsel patients of any age, and their families

- an expansion of local and national voluntary associations to provide advice and information to all patients and professionals who are involved with epilepsy

- the introduction of legal measures, including through the Disability Discrimination Act, to help ensure that individuals with epilepsy are fairly treated in employment and other areas of life.

In the authors' opinion, it will be the continuing expansion of epilepsy clinics and the appointment of nurses and appropriately trained and interested doctors, rather than the identification of new anti-epileptic drugs, that will most significantly improve the quality of life of patients who have epilepsy.

Funding for research into epilepsy

Unfortunately, many of the above facilities are not yet available due to lack of funding, the relative lack of which also affects opportunities for research, and for attracting young researchers into the field. Epilepsy is, unfortunately, not regarded as important as many other clinical disorders when it comes to allocating funds for research. With the recent development of new anti-epileptic drugs, the pharmaceutical industry has provided generous support and sponsorship, particularly in areas of patient and professional education. The National Institute for Health and Clinical Excellence (NICE) representing England and Wales and the Scottish Intercollegiate Guidelines Network (SIGN) representing Scotland, have published guidelines on how epilepsy in children and adults should be investigated and managed. This has now provided the NHS including Primary Care Trusts (PCTs), general practitioners and hospital trusts with a clearer picture of epilepsy and how patients with epilepsy should be cared for. Time (and money) will tell as to whether the NICE and SIGN guidelines have resulted in improved care for these people and their families.

Charitable organizations, often working through university departments and large epilepsy centres (Appendix 2) are other very important sources of funding for research and development. These include Epilepsy Research UK, which is the largest organization funding basic scientific and clinical research into epilepsy in the UK, and Epilepsy Action, The National Society for Epilepsy and Epilepsy Bereaved. It is also hoped that there will be increased collaboration in both clinical work and research with the rest of Europe, through the European Union, and also the United States, although such research will have to circumvent the usual bureaucracy and red tape involved in any cross-country projects.

Progress is likely to occur by the gradual accumulation of new knowledge. There are medical and scientific journals, including *Epilepsia, Epilepsy Research, Seizure, Epileptic Disorders, Epilepsy & Behavior*, as well as many other paediatric and adult neurology journals that are committed to the publication of the results of the best research in epilepsy. There are also regular regional, national, European and international meetings for all those interested and involved in epilepsy to generate ideas, collaborate in research, and then disseminate and share any advances throughout the world.

Finally, increased funding in research and the greater provision of education and services for people with epilepsy will almost certainly improve their quality of life. Additional benefits from this research will almost certainly lead to a much better understanding of epilepsy and how it affects affected individuals, and at all ages. An increased understanding in part depends upon an increased knowledge about this group of conditions, and increased knowledge, dispelling the myths and mysteries about epilepsy. We hope this book has helped to do just that.

Appendix 1

Patient perspectives

The following pieces, the first written by Sam, a teenager with epilepsy, the second written by his parents, illustrate some of the many issues that young people with epilepsy, and their families, have to face when given a diagnosis of epilepsy. These include:

- the diagnosis of epilepsy and impact this may have on the family

- the cause of epilepsy (although a tumour is a very rare cause of epilepsy in children)

- the treatment of epilepsy, the fact that some anti-epileptic drugs may have side-effects and also the role of surgery in curing some people with epilepsy

- the persisting stigma of epilepsy and how this can be addressed by the young person and their family.

Sam: 'Epilepsy for me was diagnosed at an age where I could understand the majority of it; just like most boys do at the age of 8! I wanted to have a career that would make me well known and my personal choice was to be a helicopter pilot. Of course, knowing that having epilepsy wouldn't allow such a job made me upset, but at the same time made me think of how I could help people with similar conditions a lot more easily because of the empathy we would share.

As I grew up, I learnt that the friends you hold closest to you are there for you when it all seems doom and gloom; the main reason being they don't automatically think of flashing lights at the sound of the word 'epileptic'. I don't know why there is this constant association between epilepsy and flashing lights. Instead, they open their minds past the stereotype and seem willing to learn about the different types of epilepsy. However, several years on, some people are still narrow-minded enough to believe that the stereotype is the truth.

My school life was also a little injured but despite what has happened I am striving to pass all my GCSEs with a forever thank you to my friends, family and the work that the doctors have done to help me. Along with those thanks and memories I will never forget the wise words of my mother when feeling low about having epilepsy: 'It's what you've got, not who you are'.

Sam's parents: 'During a particular parents evening at junior school, we were shocked when Sam's teacher informed us that he was not concentrating in class. She stated that he was lazy and at times appeared vacant with his mind elsewhere, and his work was not up to his usual high standards. Sam told us he was trying his best, but admitted that there were times when he did find it difficult to concentrate but couldn't explain why. Sam also mentioned that he was experiencing feelings in his head which he could only describe as 'fizzies'.

Following a couple of hospital visits we were given the possible diagnosis of epilepsy. After a number of investigations, it was thought that the epilepsy was arising from his left temporal lobe and that a brain scan had suggested this might be a brain tumour, but probably a very benign tumour. Having met with a neurologist and neurosurgeon, we were told that the most appropriate treatment would be surgery, with all the consequences that such a procedure would entail. However, whilst waiting for a repeat MRI brain scan, it was suggested that we should try to control his seizures with different anti-epileptic medication.

Following that consultation, the forty-five-minute drive home was one of the longest journeys we had ever made, we were devastated and upset as we tried to digest and comprehend what we had been told—life wasn't fair, and the tears that we shed that night were to be the first of many.

The medication that Sam was initially prescribed, whilst controlling the seizures to some degree, also had noticeable side-effects as they made him extremely drowsy, tired, and unsteady on his feet to such an extent that on one occasion he fell into someone's garden whilst walking to school. He put on a large amount of weight and suffered some of the antisocial stigma that such a complaint attracts; he was the victim of bullying at school and was actually assaulted on more than one occasion.

He became a social outcast due to the ignorance and apathy of parents of some of his school friends; he was no longer welcome at their homes, he was no longer invited to parties and was no longer asked to go for days out with them. He became listless, withdrawn and lonely, spending all of his spare time in his room, not wanting to go anywhere or do anything.

Whilst my wife and I were at work and he was at school, we used to dread the telephone ringing, as it was a frequent occurrence to hear the voice on the other end saying 'Sam is feeling unwell' or 'Sam has been sick' and there were occasions when he did in fact collapse. We would duly go and bring him home and attempt to reassure him, and each other, that he would be okay.

As a result of increased support from the medical staff and their advice, we in turn tried to educate people, including his teachers, as to how to cope with and manage Sam's ill health during such episodes. In some cases, we were successful, but there were times when it was evident that people just wanted him out of the way as his seizures were said to be disrupting the other children. However, we are of the opinion that there were times when they wanted to avoid any responsibility for his welfare.

Fortunately, his seizure control improved to the point where he was not experiencing any seizures—and he lost all the excess weight he had previously gained. However, after about fifteen months of this really good period, he began to have breakthrough seizures which continued despite an increase in medication. A repeat MRI scan revealed that the tumour had changed in appearance and characteristics although it had not grown in size.

Once again we found ourselves contemplating and fearing the prospect of surgery. When we told him, Sam was distraught, upset, and angry, and refused to listen to us, stating that he did not want to become 'a cabbage'.

We all had further discussions with both the neurologist and neurosurgeon, including the fact that surgery would be invasive and intricate. We were gently made aware of the risks that such a procedure would entail, but also the consequences to Sam if surgery was not undertaken. Sam eventually decided that he wanted the tumour removed, and this was just three months later. Twelve months following surgery, he is still seizure-free and his anti-epileptic medication is about to be withdrawn.

Sam now enjoys an excellent quality of life, and is able to do everything that an able-bodied teenager of his age should be doing; he has an active social life and is gaining excellent results in his GCSE studies. He also has developed a degree of independence that none of us thought was possible.

He represents his school at hockey, has recently been nominated for head boy, is an active member of the school council, and is a senior prefect. His educational achievements are impressive, more so when consideration is given to his absences due to his ill health and hospital appointments.

These past years have been emotionally, psychologically and physically challenging for us all, but we have experienced tremendous support from family, friends, Sam's school, our respective employers and all medical bodies concerned with his welfare.

Sam has touched many hearts with his perseverance, determination and positive attitude, and he never lost faith; his character and self belief has enabled him to overcome these difficult and trying times, with a vigour and purpose, and my wife and I are immensely proud of him.'

Appendix 2

Useful addresses (correct as of June 2008)

Brainwave

The Irish Epilepsy Association
249 Crumlin Road
Dublin 12
Ireland
Tel: 00 353 1 455 7500
Fax: 00 353 1 455 7013
Website: http://www.epilepsy.ie
E-mail: info@epilepsy.ie

Employment Medical Advisory Service

Health and Safety Executive
EMAS (London Division)
Rosecourt
2 Southwark Bridge
London SE1 9HS
HSE Infoline: 0845 345 0055
Fax: 020 7556 2109
Website: http://www.hse.gov.uk

Driver and Vehicle Licensing Agency

Longview Road
Swansea SA6 7JL
Tel: 01792 782341
Website: http://www.dvla.gov.uk

Epilepsy Action (formerly British Epilepsy Association)

New Anstey House
Gateway Drive
. Yeadon
Leeds LS19 7XY
Tel: 0113 210 8800
Fax: 0113 391 0300
Helpline: Freephone 0808 800 5050
Website: http://www.epilepsy.org.uk
E-mail: epilepsy@epilepsy.org.uk
International Helpline: +44 113 210 8800

Epilepsy Bereaved

PO Box 112
Wantage
Oxon, OX12 8XT
Tel/Fax: 01235 772 850
Bereavement Contact Line: 01235 772852
Website: http://www.sudep.org
E-mail: epilepsybereaved@org.uk

Epilepsy Action Scotland

48 Govan Road
Glasgow G51 1JL
Tel: 0141 427 4911
Fax: 0141 419 1709
Website: http://www.epilepsyscotland.org.uk
E-mail: enquiries@epilepsyscotland.org.uk
Helpline: 0808 800 2200

Epilepsy Wales

PO Box 4168
Cardiff

CF14 OWZ
Helpline: 0845 741 3774
Website: http://www.epilepsy-wales.co.uk
E-mail: office@epilepsy-wales.co.uk
Admin tel.: 02920 755515
Fax: 02920 755515
E-mail: webmaster@epilepsy-wales.co.uk
E-mail: admin@epilepsy-wales.co.uk

Epilepsy Canada

2255B Queen Street E,
Suite 336
Toronto, Ontario
M4E 1G3
Canada.
Toll Free 1-877-734-0873
Tel: 001 514 845 7855
Website: http://www.epilepsy.ca
E-mail: epilepsy@epilepsy.ca

Epilepsy Foundation of America

8301 Professional Place
Landover MD20785
USA
Tel: 001 800 332 1000
Website: http://www.epilepsyfoundation.org

Epilepsy Research UK

PO Box 3004
London W4 1XT
Tel/Fax: 0208 995 4781
Website: http://www.epilepsyresearch.org.uk

International Bureau for Epilepsy

IBE

Achterweg 5

2103 SW Heemstede

The Netherlands

Tel: 0031 235 291019

E-mail: ibe@xs4all.nl.

MedicAlert

No. 1 Bridge Wharf

156 Caledonian Road,

London, N1 9UU

Free Phone 0800 581420

Tel: 020 7833 3034

Website: http://www.medicalert.org.uk

E-mail: info@medicalert.org.uk

Mersey Regional Epilepsy Association

Neuro Support Centre

Norton Street

Liverpool, L3 8LR

Tel: 0151 298 2666

Fax: 0151 298 2333

Website: http://www.epilepsymersey.org.uk

E-mail: epilepsy@mrea.demon.co.uk

National Society for Epilepsy

Chesham Lane

Chalfont St Peter

Buckinghamshire SL9 ORJ

Tel: 01494 601300

Fax: 01494 871927

Helpline: 01494 601400

Website: http://www.epilepsynse.org.uk

Index